CHANGE OF HEART
Never Lose Hope

LIESL SCHOONRAAD-
GREGORY

© Liesl Schoonraad 2022
www.usa-hope.com
ISBN: 9798353358794

All rights reserved. No part of this publication may be reproduced, distributed, or transmitted in any form or by any means, including photocopying, recording, or other electronic or mechanical methods, without the prior written permission of the publisher, except in the case of brief quotations embodied in critical reviews and certain other non-commercial use permitted by copyright law.

Ezekiel 36:26

I will give you a new heart and put a new spirit in you; I will remove from you your heart of stone and give you a heart of flesh.

DEDICATION

This book is dedicated to Deedra Marie Manning. You had an appointment with God on a tragic day, but you left the ultimate gift of hope, saving my husband.

To Dee's family, we will always be connected through Dee's Heart.

We will continue to celebrate her life.

ALL THE GLORY TO GOD! Our promise keeper. Our miracle worker. Our way maker.

ACKNOWLEDGEMENT

Thank you to Dr. Masashi Kai, Dr. Avi Levine, Dr. Gregg Lanier, and the entire Heart Team as well as every single member of the staff at Westchester Medical Center in New York. You have touched more than our lives, you have touched our souls.

Thank you to Harboring Hearts for your incredible support through this challenging journey. You were light during a very dark time.

Thank you to Anna Lisa Vitale and Ashleigh Voros, @SplitLeafSaturdays, for your incredible guidance and support as Editors of this book.

Thank you to my husband, Stan. You have been through so much and yet you shine. God is not done with you yet.

Most of all, thank you, Papa, Jesus. Thank you for this journey, this rollercoaster. Thank you for the lessons, the miracles, and the experience. Thank you for showing us, firsthand, what HOPE is and never giving up on us. Amen.

INTRODUCTION

I have been an organ donor for many years but until the winter of 2021 I never fully understood the incredible gift one can leave behind for others. They say you never understand a journey until you have traveled it. I have found this to be ultimately true.

We never know how strong we are until we need to be. Sometimes it feels like the challenge is too much to bear but the strength of the human spirit is incredible.

Never give up hope! You never know if a miracle is awaiting you. Keep going. No matter how hard it might feel.

Somehow we made it through and I look back and wonder, how did I do it? Yet, I did. We did.

In the fall of 2021, my husband and I were about to go on a roller coaster ride. There was no stopping this ride and we never chose to take this ride but sometimes "life" happens and we find ourselves having to deal with whatever knocks us down.

Jesus take the wheel. We are about to go on a journey which will change our lives completely.

This is a true story of how there is hope even in the darkness. Proof we should never give up and, most of all, how God performs miracles. All we have to do is surrender to Him.

CONTENTS

Chapter 1	A Failing Heart	19
Chapter 2	God's Promise	75
Chapter 3	Blind Faith	87
Chapter 4	Setbacks and Blessings	123
Chapter 5	Thanksgiving	167
Chapter 6	Total Surrender	179
Chapter 7	Miracles	199
Chapter 8	Touched by An Angel	219
Chapter 9	Delirium	243
Chapter 10	Healing	265
Chapter 11	A Christmas Miracle	271
Chapter 12	Losing Dave Maroney	279
Chapter 13	Her name was Deedra	287

MUSIC PLAYLIST

I decided to add a music playlist to the book. These songs inspired and uplifted me during this journey.

- "Tell Your Heart To Beat Again" - Danny Gokey
- "While I wait" – Lincoln Brewster
- "Waymaker" - Leeland
- "I Surrender" - Hillsong Worship
- "I Am Not Alone" - Kari Jobe
- "I Need You" - Chris Tomlin
- "Run TO THe Father" - Cody Carnes
- "Goodness Of God" - TRIBL & Mav City Music
- "You're Gonna Be Okay" - Brian & Jenn Johnson
- "Even When It Hurts" - Hillsong United
- "Ocean Spirit Lead Me" - Hillsong United
- "It Is Well" - Kristene DiMarco
- "Amazing Grace" - Royal Scots Dragoon Guards

PROLOGUE

I met my husband Stan through a mutual friend on Facebook in 2017. I was living in Cape Town, South Africa and he lived in Upstate New York in the USA.

We never spoke in private till late 2017 when I messaged him for the first time. I wanted to tell him how much I enjoyed his humor. I always believed that giving compliments was important and that was exactly what my intention was sending a message to Stan.

Stan of course, tells a different story of how I stalked him, and never left him alone. All ego talk.

From that day, our messages turned into voice messages and into phone calls. We have a lot in common. Stan was a building contractor and I had originally studied Architecture. We were both powerlifters and then there was the humor.

In July of 2018 Stan sent me a message that read, "I just emailed God".

I smiled and responded, "You have His email address?" What did you say?"

"I asked Him why he dropped you thousands of miles away from me," he replied.

"Well, let me know when you get a reply," I laughed.

We decided that maybe we should meet face to face and during the fall of 2018 I spent five weeks here in the USA with Stan. We were keen to continue a relationship but I was way too independent to even consider a, *have to get married in 90 days,* type of visa.

Due to the work I did in South Africa I managed to qualify for a Visa for Person with Extraordinary Ability and would be able to work in schools and with veterans here in the USA.

When I flew back to South Africa, I heard God speak to me and say, "You need to go home and sell everything, you are not going to move back to South Africa again".

God had a plan and when He has a plan things run smoothly. And it did. Within three months my visa application was approved, a process that normally takes up to a year or even longer.

I had sold everything, said goodbye to friends and family, and found myself on an airplane back to JFK Airport. From JFK I would take a connecting flight to Rochester.

When I touched down in Rochester I became emotional. It felt like I was a little homesick already, yet I just arrived home.

It was a massive adjustment to move countries, traumatizing in many ways, but this is where God wanted me to be.

On September 26, 2020, Stan and I got married. I became a permanent US Resident. I was looking forward to a lifetime here in the USA with Stan, but my journey was about to take a huge detour.

CHAPTER 1

A Failing Heart

A roller-coaster ride. That is how I would describe where our lives were heading. We didn't get onto this ride by choice. Life happened. God had a plan.

"God give me strength," I would pray.

Well, God was about to give it to me. But to get stronger, we need to go through challenges. Be careful what you pray for, you might just get it!

We would experience ups and downs like never before. The scary moments and the close calls. The incredible adrenaline rushes, and wondering if this ride would ever end.

Let's start at the beginning.

I was driving alone, my packed bags on the back seat. The roads were exceptionally quiet, even for 3 a.m. The darkness surrounded me.

Fall leaves kept dropping on the road ahead. A deer froze on the side of the road, caught in my headlights. I had no time to slow down, I needed to get to New York City. Our eyes locked till I passed him.

Would Stan still be alive when I get there? Would I be in time to say goodbye? My thoughts were racing and passed me at 65 miles per hour. "NO! Jesus you PROMISED me!

I am keeping to your promise Papa. You are not the type of Father who has brought us this far and to drop us now. Please PAPA!" I was in constant prayer.

The rhythmic sound of the tires over the cracks in the road reminded me of Stan's racing heart monitor in the background on the phone…

The enemy knew, my Achilles heel was my mind. It always tried to mess with my mind to veer me off course. If I kept speaking to Papa, my head would clear and I would again feel my faith growing. The enemy was NOT going to win this battle!

I kept checking the GPS to see how long till I reached Westchester Medical Center. I had four hours remaining. "PLEASE PLEASE Papa," I cried out once more and I wiped my eyes quickly with the palm of my hand as I struggled to see through the tears building up.

I took a few deeper breaths and opened the window a little more. The cool air through my hair felt refreshing. But like the window opened wider the enemy was working on opening my mind to its lies. After all, that's its job, to kill, steal and destroy.

"NO! Papa, help me, help Stan. PLEASE Papa, I am not ready to be a widow. We haven't even celebrated our second wedding anniversary. Jesus you promised, I am holding onto the promise right now, like never before. I KNOW You are going to come through for us! Please forgive me for doubting your promise Papa," I kept praying every time I felt the enemy draw closer but it felt like it was attacking me from all sides.

Maybe it was easier in the dark.

I moved my eyes to the side of the road for a quick second and all I could see was forest, trees everywhere. Then the light would disappear and there was just darkness. When I looked back to the road ahead, all I could focus on was the yellow line on the road, fading into the darkness ahead.

This was what my faith now became. Blind faith. Believing God knows the road ahead even though I could not see it beyond where the light caught it. I had to believe the road continued for me and Stan.

I continued driving, no idea where this journey was taking me, but having faith that Jesus was going to allow me to find my husband alive when I got to the hospital. He promised!

Maybe I should go back a little further and start at the very beginning.

Tuesday, November 9, 2021

It was a beautiful early fall morning. Beautifully colored autumn leaves dropped slowly outside our bedroom window.

Boat owners started lifting their boat launches from the lake as the snow season drew closer. The smell of cinnamon and spice hung in the air as we started to celebrate fall.

Stan was fast asleep. He was recovering from a concrete job he completed the previous week. He has been a concrete mason most of his life, a job not many can do, especially for the amount of years Stan put in.

"Not for the faint of heart" many would say, but there he was, a man with heart failure and still doing concrete work.

He used to be able to bounce back quicker after a big job but over the past three years, I could see he needed more and more time to recover.

It was not surprising. Stan had been suffering from heart failure for more than fifteen years and what used to come easy and natural to him was becoming harder and harder to accomplish.

With medication and regular checkups, he was able to keep going but I could see a faster deterioration happening.

He was hospitalized in late August of 2021 for almost 3 weeks and his heart failure medications were pushed to the maximum.

I reached over and gently placed my hand on his chest. I could feel his failing heart beating. He slowly opened his eyes and put his hand on top of mine. "Good morning beautiful," Stan said and closed his eyes again.

"Good morning. How are you feeling?" I asked while gently rubbing his chest.

"Tired," he responded. He hardly managed to open his eyes.

"Sleep a little more, I will go get breakfast started, okay?" I said as I got up. I pulled the covers over him making sure he was warm. One could feel the change of season in the air.

"Sounds good," Stan replied and dozed off again.

Walking to the kitchen I wondered if I should try and call the doctor again, but it seemed they did everything they could for him when he was in the hospital a few months earlier.

Since he had come home from this last hospital visit, he was struggling with stomach pains and the doctors just couldn't figure out what was happening other than his heart was weakening.

It's strange sometimes how we refuse to see the inevitable. A form of denial, I suppose. The fact was, his heart was failing fast and we didn't want to see the reality of it.

We didn't want to see that this was not going to get better. It was about to get worse, much worse.

As I opened the fridge door and took the eggs and milk out I heard Stan getting up and going into the bathroom.

I had a moment of relief knowing he was up but it was short-lived as I heard him get sick. I ran over to the bathroom and found the door ajar.

I peeked in. He was folded over the basin rinsing his mouth. "Honey, are you okay?" I asked and he slowly stood up.

"I am SO tired, Liesl, and my stomach is killing me," Stan replied. He had a look of desperation on his face and his eyes had lost their sparkle.

"This is ridiculous, these doctors need to figure this out. I am going to call the office again," I said and walked to the kitchen to call the doctor's office.

Stan went back to bed. He could hardly keep his eyes open.

I dialed the doctor's office and got annoyed with the three minutes of COVID 19 messages before a human finally answered the phone.

"Good morning, how can we help you," a voice answered.

"Hi. This is Mrs. Gregory and I need to speak to the doctor about my husband Stan Gregory. He is not well and his stomach is not getting any better. When are we going to get this referral done for the specialist? This has taken way too long," I demanded.

"I am sorry Mrs. Gregory that it is taking so long but I can give you their number then maybe you can call them and explain the urgency?" the nurse replied.

Why it suddenly became my job - I do not know, but I needed to start taking action. I became my husband's advocate, not realizing how important this advocacy was going to become.

She continued to give me the specialist's number. I called their office and when the receptionist answered I was immediately on her case.

"Good morning. This is Mrs. Gregory, Stan Gregory's wife. My husband's primary has been trying to get a referral to you for weeks now. My husband needs to make an appointment urgently please, he is NOT well," I said, trying my best to stay calm.

"I am sorry about that, Mrs. Gregory. We can fit your husband in on December 21st if that would work for you?" the nurse replied. I was about to fume.

This was more than a month away and there was no way my husband was going to make it waiting that long.

"Nevermind, thank you, I will take him to the emergency department later today," I said.

"I am sorry about that Mrs. Gregory," the nurse said with almost no compassion in her voice.

I hung up and walked to the bedroom. Stan was resting and still found it hard to simply open his eyes. I sat on the bed next to him and placed my hand on his shoulder.

"Honey, the specialist cannot see you until late December. I think it's time we go back to the emergency department. Why don't you take a shower and let me take you?" I suggested.

"I guess that's what we will have to do. I will get up in a minute," Stan mumbled.

For about three hours I kept nagging at him to get up until I threatened to call 911. He simply didn't have the energy to get up and go. As he realized I was about to call an ambulance, he finally pushed himself to take a quick shower.

As we drove to the city, about thirty minutes away, I explained to Stan to keep his phone and charger close as I won't be able to go into the emergency department with him.

The hospitals didn't allow anyone but the patient into the ED due to COVID. He agreed and said he would call me once he has any feedback but I should probably go home as he thinks it might be a few hours.

I knew it might be more than a few hours, maybe a few days. I drove home with a heavy heart. My gut said there was about to be a tough road ahead, but I would never have guessed how tough.

Later that afternoon, I found myself staring out the kitchen window for a while with a cup of coffee in my hand, watching the autumn leaves fall. Squirrels running frantically to collect their last winter stash. They had no care in the world.

I had lost track of time when my phone rang. It startled me and I nearly spilled my coffee. I grabbed at the phone on the kitchen counter. It was Stan.

"Hey honey, what's happening?" I asked quickly.

"Hey. Not too sure yet. They did some tests, going to do more and also do some more blood tests. The doctor thinks it's my heart causing the stomach issues," Stan said with a weak but clear voice.

"It sounds like you are at least being taken care of right now, that's good. We will take it one step at a time, right?" I replied.

"All we can do, yes, I will call you later if I have more news. I am just resting and waiting," Stan said.

"Sounds good. I love you," I said. "Love you too, Honey, I'll call you later," Stan said and hung up.

At that very moment, I knew. I knew this was the end of more than fifteen years of heart failure. Stan's heart was running on fumes and struggling.

I phoned Stan's brother, Stewart, or Stew, like Stan calls him, to let him know what was happening and promised to keep him updated. I didn't want to call anyone else as I thought I would prefer to do so when I have more information as to what exactly was happening.

As I sat down on the couch, I started praying. "Lord Jesus, I need You right now. Stan needs You right now. Papa, I cannot do this alone. I need You to help me and guide me. Please, Papa," I prayed.

Wednesday, November 10, 2021

I fell asleep while praying and crying. At one o'clock in the morning, the sudden ringing of my telephone woke me up. It was a Rochester General Hospital phone number. This could not be good…

It is amazing how fast the mind works. In that split second before answering I thought, why is Stan not calling me? Why is the hospital calling me? This really cannot be good.

"Hello?" I answered quickly.

"Is this Mrs. Gregory speaking?" the male voice asked.

"Yes, it is." I replied.

"Mrs. Gregory, this is Dr. Hussein from the Rochester General Hospital. I just called you to bring you up to date about your husband, Stan Gregory. We have moved your husband to the Cardiac ICU. Mrs. Gregory, your husband is very ill," the doctor explained.

"What exactly is going on doctor?" I asked.

"Your husband's heart is struggling, Mrs. Gregory. His organs are in failure due to a lack of blood supply. His heart is simply not strong enough to feed the organs with enough blood supply, so the kidneys and liver are also struggling and busy failing," the doctor continued.

My world as I knew it was about to collapse and I couldn't find words.

"Can you do anything for him?" I asked.

"Currently we are doing more tests and giving him what we can to support his heart. Will you be coming to see him in the morning?" the doctor asked.

"Absolutely yes. What time can I see him?" I asked.

"Visiting hours start at 9 am. If you can be here around that time I can explain more as I will have more information by then," Doctor Hussein said.

"Thank you, doctor, I will see you at 9 am. Thank you," I said and cannot even remember if I said goodbye as reality hit me like a ton of bricks.

I didn't want to call Stewart at 1 a.m. as there wasn't anything he could do and I didn't have all the info yet. I spent the rest of the early morning in prayer on my couch. Crying. Trying my best to stay strong.

Ironic how I used to be a Strongwoman, pulling trucks for sport, but this was a different kind of strength and I was not sure I was strong enough to finish this challenge. There was no other option. I HAD to be strong.

Just like pulling a truck, trying to do the impossible, I had to do the same now. Not focus on the task or how heavy the load is, but rather on keeping my head down, believing anything is possible.

Taking small steps, not looking how far I need to go but rather focusing on each little step and believing each step brings me closer to the destination. No matter how much it hurts, no matter how many times the enemy screams in my ear, "this is impossible", to ignore the negative and to keep going. I had to keep believing that the impossible is possible.

"Hold my hand once more Papa, I need to walk this road of impossibility again, I cannot do it without You," I prayed.

I was first in line at the Hospital reception waiting to sign in as a visitor at 9 a.m. All the standard COVID questions and temperature were taken.

"Mr. Gregory is in room 2003 in the Cardiac ICU on the second floor," the friendly lady said and handed me a sticker for identification.

Frantically, I worked my way to the ICU and was met at reception by a very friendly voice. I hated not being able to see people's smiles with the masks on their faces.

"Good morning. Who are you here to visit today?" she asked.

"My husband, Stan Gregory, I believe he is in room 2003," I replied and she handed me a gown wrapped in plastic.

She smiled and said, "Mrs. Gregory, you can put this gown on over your clothing and find a pair of gloves at the door, the doctor will be with you shortly."

Why must I wear a gown? Gloves? What's going on? So many questions ran through my mind but I kept focus on the instructions.

I could see Stan through the glass window at the end of the hallway. He was sleeping and a nurse was working on his IV bags.

As I got to the door I put my handbag down. I dressed in the gown and took a pair of gloves from the cart at the door.

The nurse noticed me, walked over, and asked, "Mrs. Gregory?"

"Yes, morning, how is my husband?" I replied.

"He is very tired, but stable. The doctor is around and I am sure he will come to update you. You are welcome to come in and speak to your husband."

I walked over to Stan's bedside, overwhelmed by all the IV lines, but mostly by how tired he looked. His color seemed off. I had never seen him look like this before.

I leaned down slowly and kissed him on the forehead.

"Hey, you. I'm here," I said and he slowly opened his eyes.

"Morning, honey," Stan said softly.

Two doctors entered the room and I walked over, closer to them.

"Mrs. Gregory, I am Dr. Hussein. I spoke to you early this morning," the one doctor said.

"Morning doctor, how is my husband doing?" I asked.

"He is struggling, Mrs. Gregory. We are still awaiting some test results but I might need to ask your consent for a procedure later depending on the results," Dr. Hussein explained.

"What kind of procedure?" I asked.

"It is called an IABP. Simply put, a balloon pump. We place a balloon pump into the artery that takes blood from the heart to the rest of the body to help the blood pump stronger," Dr. Hussein continued to explain.

"Does he need open heart surgery for that?" I asked.

"No, we place the pump through the groin but it is done under anesthesia in the OR," Dr. Hussein said with a concerned look.

"And that will help? That will be the answer to him getting better?" I asked.

"It is the best thing we can do for him right now but it is not a permanent solution. Right now we have to take things one step at a time and this will be our first step to try and get Mr. Gregory as stable as possible," Dr. Hussein said.

"Will you be around to sign some paperwork later if needed? Your husband is simply too tired and I tried to explain this to him earlier but he fell asleep while I explained," Dr. Hussein said with a slight grin.

"Yes, I will be here all day. I will be at the cafeteria during lunch when there are no visiting hours, but I will be around, whatever you need I will sign," I said.

"Thank you, Mrs. Gregory. I will be in touch as soon as we get more results. I have your number if I need to call you," Dr. Hussein tried to give a reassuring nod and left the room.

I walked over to Stan and I could feel my heart get heavy. Since I met Stan, I was always the positive one and now was the time to prove I can always find the positivity, no matter how hard, but this was tough.

Facing the unknown is always hard and this is where "blind faith" comes in. Having faith that God is in control when you cannot see the outcome. Believing He is in total control of the situation and that He has a plan.

The nurse brought me a chair and I pulled it as close as I could to the bedside to hold Stan's hand without interfering with any of the medical equipment. I just sat there.

Silently praying for hours, having a spiritual battle to remain in faith and not succumb to the negative thoughts the enemy tried to throw at me.

I stepped aside and called Stewart explaining that the doctor asked me to sign permission for them to possibly do the procedure later in the day.

We agreed that there was not much choice and that they needed to do whatever they could to help Stan. It was a relief to have Stewart to support me with decisions as we're both Stan's proxies but more importantly, family.

The nurse was with Stan almost all the time and so many different doctors came in and out of the room over the next few hours.

A doctor from disease control came in to ask a bunch of questions as they were still making sure his stomach issue was not due to some disease or bacteria not related to the heart. Now I understood the whole gown and gloves dress code.

I knew however, this was not the problem. Stan had been sick for weeks and if it was contagious I would have been sick by this time, but I was fine. There was no doubt in my mind it was all heart-related.

If the heart could not pump enough blood to the kidneys and liver, I am sure his stomach was also struggling. It now made sense why his stomach was hurting so bad after he ate. There would not be enough blood supply to help the stomach digest the food, causing pain.

I was staring out the window at the beautiful colors of the turning leaves of the trees in the car park when Dr. Hussein walked into the room.

"Mrs. Gregory. We got some results back and we will have to continue with the Balloon Pump as explained. Unfortunately, his numbers are looking worse and have not improved with the medications," the doctor said.

"Anything he needs, doctor. Whatever I need to sign. When will he have this procedure?" I asked.

"Now. We need to help his heart as quickly as we can," he said trying to reassure me, but I could see the concern in his eyes.

"Thank you, doctor, thank you," I said, struggling not to burst into tears.

Minutes later the OR staff walked in and said they were there to take Stan for his surgery.

I kissed Stan on the forehead and said, "I love you."

The reality hit me that this could be the last time.

He was so weak. What if he didn't make it through the surgery? The enemy was messing with my mind again.

The surgeon came into the room and explained he will be doing the procedure and would call me the moment he is done. He recommended I go get some coffee as it would take a while.

I watched as they wheeled my husband out of the room. Surrounded by doctors, nurses and students. I stood there in the room. Alone. Trying to keep it together, and I did. But only till I got to the car.

I broke down and had a good cry before I took a deep breath and googled where I could get some coffee and find a park to sit for a while.

I watched my phone like a hawk. It felt like days had passed but it was only a few hours until I got the call.

"Mrs. Gregory, the surgery went well and your husband is in recovery. He did very well and I am sure his kidney and liver numbers will improve. You are welcome to come and see him in about an hour," the surgeon explained.

"Thank you so, so much doctor. Thank you," I said feeling incredibly relieved at the moment.

I was not prepared for what I saw when I walked back into Stan's room. He had an IV line in his neck called a Central Line. A machine standing next to his bed making pumping sounds with something that looked like another heart monitor. It was the balloon pump.

Not a single heartbeat looked the same. The pumping sounds were irregular. The machine struggled to find a rhythm to support the heart. There was a full leg brace on Stan's right leg from his ankle to his groin with wires coming out the top. It prevented him from moving and interfering with the balloon pump access.

There were seven or more IV bags on a stand next to him running through a fusion machine controlling how much of each medication is dispensed. All the tubes running to the Central Line.

I pulled up a chair and gently put my hand inside Stan's hand and just sat there. Staring at all the equipment. The reality of how sick he was hit me once again. Like a swinging punching bag. Just as you get your breath back it hits you from behind.

It felt like hours had passed but the clock on the wall ticked by slowly. Second by second. The doctor walked in and, once again, had a concerned look on his face.

"Mrs. Gregory, your husband has stabilized but not improved. We will have to place an Impella Heart pump through the chest below the collar bone to assist his heart better if things do not improve in the next few hours," he explained.

"Another pump?" I asked, confused. "This will replace the balloon. It will be able to pump the blood out of the heart better. I suggest we do the procedure this evening," the doctor said.

"Tonight?" I asked in disbelief.

"Yes. I will need your signature again and I will call you once surgery has been completed," he said.

They managed to get Stan into surgery earlier than planned. The doctor suggested I go home and come in to see him the following morning.

Driving home, I remember watching people pass me on the freeway and I had a strange thought. The world keeps going no matter what life-changing experience we are having.

It felt like the world was moving past me while I was frozen in time.

When I got home, I made myself a cup of coffee and sat down on the couch to call our family and friends. It was mentally exhausting to repeat myself and I got lost in whom I updated on what but I felt the support and care from loved ones.

I sat back and once again, tears started flowing.

"Lord Jesus, please help me, please help Stan. Help us cope with this process, Lord," I prayed.

That night, I felt a sense of peace settle over me.

Thursday, November 11, 2021

I hated being late for things; I was again the first person in line the following morning for visiting hours. I didn't want to miss a single moment I could be with Stan.

As I walked into the Cardiac ICU, the receptionist greeted me and said they moved Stan to another room. They had cleared Stan of any infectious disease which meant I didn't need a gown.

As I walked into the room, I was expecting to see a sleeping Stan but was pleasantly surprised by him being wide awake.

"Good morning honey," Stan said with a sound of renewed life in his voice.

Something I had not heard for some time. He was definitely feeling better.

"Hey handsome, what's up?" I said walking over to kiss him.

"I am a little upset with you," Stan replied.

I was quite taken aback when I realized he was being serious and not kidding around.
"Why? What did I do?" I was puzzled.

"You gave them permission for this procedure now there is no turning back," Stan said.

That was the first experience of a kind of delirium I would see from Stan.

"It was not an option, it was the only thing to do. You would have died without it!" I explained.

I was blown away by the fact that he was complaining that I saved his life by giving consent.

He seemed to be more accepting of my choice to let him have the procedure when the doctor walked in and said, "You obviously needed that surgery, Mr. Gregory. Your numbers look much better this morning and you are awake!" the doctor said.

"What is the next step doc?" I asked.

"I was explaining to your husband a few minutes ago that we had two options but it seems we now only have one option after looking at the results a little closer," the doctor said.

"What do you mean "had" two options and now only one, what options?" I asked.
"The one option would have been to put an LVAD in for your husband. An external heart pump that he will have until he gets a heart transplant but his heart is too weak for an LVAD, in my opinion, so I would say the other option is a transplant and it is the ONLY option," the doctor explained.

Those words hit me in my gut. Hearing the ONLY option is a heart transplant. It is amazing how the mind runs ahead and I found myself speaking my mind out loud.

"What are his chances of getting a heart? He is going to be 65 in a few days," I heard myself say.

"Again, Mrs. Gregory, we take it one step at a time. We are busy speaking to the insurance company to see if they will approve a flight for your husband to Westchester Medical Center so they can do an evaluation to be listed. We are also in contact with WMC to see if they can accept your husband for an evaluation," the doctor explained.

Overwhelm. That's the word I felt at that moment. Where is Westchester Medical Center? What do you mean evaluated? Fly down? Can I fly down with him? I had so many questions.

"I am going to send the social worker to answer any questions you might have but let's get those approvals today, ok?" the doctor said.

"Thank you doctor," I said looking over at Stan who had a look of concern, yet calm on his face.

That was normal for Stan when the wind was taken out of his sails. Like a deer in headlights. Frozen.

The doctor left the room and Stan looked over at me as I walked closer to him.

"This is serious honey, what are we going to do?" Stan asked.

"We are going to let God take control and take it a step at a time. That's what we are going to do. You are going to have to trust in God that He has your back and trust me to take care of things the best I can. You simply rest and work on getting better. I will make a plan with everything, it will all work out," I said trying to reassure myself and not just Stan.

A lady walked into the room and introduced herself as the social worker.

My first question was, "Where is Westchester located?"

"Just outside of New York City", she said.

The next questions running through my mind were, where will I stay? But most importantly, how long will we be staying?

So many questions. "Could I come and see you in a little while with my list of questions? Maybe take some notes?" I asked the social worker.

She seemed relieved at my suggestion as she must have noticed my mind was moving into overdrive. NYC is considered one of the world's top tourist attractions but now I am going to visit it for the first time under horrible circumstances.

There was one other option rather than flying Stan to Westchester. Another local hospital in Rochester did heart transplants but we knew Stan's chances of receiving a donor heart in a more populated area like NYC would be much greater for survival. A horrible reality, where there is more death there is a bigger chance of receiving a heart.

Stan looked at me concerned.

I leaned over and grabbed him by the cheeks, "It will be fine, we will work this out, focus on YOU," I said.

The doctor walked back into the room with a smile, followed by the social worker. The smile gave me a moment of hope.

"I have some good news. The insurance has approved the flight and Westchester has accepted you, Mr. Gregory," the doctor said.

"When does he fly?" I asked.

"Tomorrow at 11 am. So Mrs. Gregory, why don't you come in at 8 a.m.? I will arrange for you to come in a little earlier to spend some time with your husband before he flies?" the doctor suggested compassionately.

"Thank you, doctor, I appreciate that," I said and felt Stan taking my hand.

I felt this was yet another moment of favor from God allowing me to spend some extra time with Stan even though it was against hospital policy.

"Doctor, is this the route you would choose if Stan was your brother?" I asked, wanting a final word of confirmation.

"Most definitely, without a doubt," the doctor replied with great understanding on his face.
"I will see you in a little while, Mrs. Gregory?" the social worker asked with a smile.

"Yes, thank you!" I replied.

Stan and I found ourselves alone in the room for the first time. I leaned closer to his face.

"God is going to get you through this," I said as I looked deep into his eyes.

"I hope so," Stan replied. "I KNOW so," I said with reassurance.

"Are you going to come down to the hospital?" Stan asked.

"OF COURSE! Stanley Harold Gregory! Monday is your birthday and I won't miss it for the world!" I said with a smile.

"I will be here with you till you fly out tomorrow. Then I will pack and sort everything at the house, have the car's wheel noise fixed and drive down Monday morning early so I can be there with you. Okay?" I said.

I wanted Stan to feel reassured of my support.

"Sounds good honey. Will you be ok driving down?" Stan asked.

"I will be just fine. I will get all the details from the social worker during lunch and you will see me there the moment visiting hours start," I said trying to reassure Stan further.

Stan is a man of few words and I felt a warmth realizing he was worried about me during a time like this.

I had no problem taking the six hour drive by myself. When I lived in South Africa, I often drove miles by myself to visit schools across the country where I did public speaking. Besides, I would have a GPS in the car and God at my side.

After a few minutes I noticed Stan fell asleep again. I sat with him, I didn't want to leave his side.

I googled where Westchester Medical Center is and looked at their website. I was disappointed to see their visiting hours are only from 2-6 p.m. due to COVID and not from 9 a.m. to 1 p.m. and 3-7 p.m. like at Rochester General Hospital.

I told myself I would spend the mornings sorting out all the daily, weekly, and monthly personal things via telephone and see Stan in the afternoon for the full visiting hours.

Then, another ton of bricks hit me as I continued reading visiting restrictions. 'All visitors need to be fully vaccinated and show proof thereof or have a negative COVID PCR test taken within the last 5 days to be able to enter the hospital.' I could not believe what I was reading.

We were not vaccinated as we had heard of people who had cardiac issues after the vaccine. Seeing as Stan was already struggling with a weak heart, we did not want to take the risk of him taking a final knock from the vaccine.

For myself, I am not very pro-vaccine. I always seem to end up with the full version of whatever I just vaccinated myself for within a few days.

I would end up with full-blown COVID if I got the vaccine and I would then expose Stan to it so it was not an option for me. I was not willing to go live with someone else for quarantine and expose them to it either.

A negative PCR test would be the only thing I could do. I HAD to see him on his birthday and be able to continue seeing him.

Math became my friend trying to figure out when I need to do a test, allowing time for the result but also keeping in mind the test had to be taken within five days and not forgetting most labs don't take tests over weekends.

It was also a time where *everyone* was being tested, as fear seemed to have captivated the country. If you had a runny nose, you thought you had COVID and got tested for the heck of it.

"Oh Lord, where do I go for this? What should I do?" I started praying silently.

Within five minutes of my prayer, a doctor walked into Stan's room introducing himself to me, "Morning, I am one of the doctors on the floor and I just wanted to come and say how happy I am to hear Stan is going to WMC."

He had a big smile on his face and it felt like a breath of fresh air walking into the room.

This was possibly one of my first Angel experiences on this journey.
"Good morning doctor, we are so grateful for everything you are all doing for Stan, thank you!" I replied.

"Doctor, do you know of a place nearby I would be able to do a PCR test by tomorrow so I can see Stan at WMC on Monday? I need to have a test result from a test no longer than five days prior. I don't even know where to go?" I pleaded for guidance.

"Absolutely! There is a place across the road from us. You can just walk in and ask them. They do not need appointments," he replied with a smile.

It felt like a mountain was lifted off my shoulders.

"Thank you!" I replied and he nodded. "Wishing you both all the best. You are going to be in excellent hands," he said as he walked out.

If I did the test on Friday evening after Stan was airlifted, or even Saturday morning, I should have the result by Monday and be able to see him. I would then figure out where to go in the city for the next test.

I spent an hour or so with the social worker who gave me a printout of local hotels close to the hospital, a map and address of the hospital as well as contact people's names at the hospital. It made me feel like I had a sense of control in a very out-of-control situation.

Stan and I spent the afternoon planning things I needed to do at the house before I left. I was not so familiar with snow seasons yet and winterizing the house was an unknown process to me.

He dozed off a few times but I used the time to take his calls and explain to clients what was happening and they were free to call me anytime.

I texted family members and a few close friends. It is in times like this that you realize who your true friends are. My dear friend Lisa came to my rescue with a ride back home when I needed to drop the car off at the service station. Later that day another friend, Joanie, gave me a ride back to the service station again. Suddenly I was forced to reach out for help with Stan not around and each time I would call someone for something, they were there without hesitation.

By evening I left Stan just before visiting hours were over and I drove home with a sense of overwhelm yet peace. I knew Stan was in God's hands. It was a different cry I had on the way home. Less hysterical, I guess, more of a download of emotion.

The past few days were a lot to absorb and I still had no idea what lay ahead.

I went to bed falling asleep while praying. Exhaustion knocked me out. Emotional exhaustion I had never felt before.

Friday, November 12, 2021

The next morning I was at Stan's bedside by 8 a.m. Yup, loyalty is one of my top five values.

There was excitement in the air. The nurse said he had never had a patient who was airlifted before so this was new to him and he was excited for Stan and this new experience.

By 9 a.m. we kept watching the helipad outside the window to see if we could see the helicopter come in. By 9:30 a.m. the nurse came into the room with a look of disappointment.

"I just called WMC for an update on the ETA and they said there is a storm in the city. They wanted us to follow up again at 11 a.m. to see how the weather is doing," he explained.

It meant I had more time with Stan before he left but we were also keen on getting him to WMC as soon as possible as we wanted the process of evaluation to commence.

We didn't have much time alone though. There were doctors and nurses constantly coming in to check on him. The Impella pump monitor needed to be checked to make sure there was enough Heparin to avoid blood clots from forming, his heart rhythm, blood pressure, temperature, levels in the IV bags, oxygen levels, urine output and color, the list continues.

Stan seemed in a positive mood and this helped me a lot to stay strong for him in return. Reality was not our friend and we could not ignore the fact that he was going to be airlifted soon. I kept praying God would keep him until I could see him again on Monday. Oh me of little faith!

Time ticked by. At 11 a.m. the nurse called again and they confirmed they would be there to collect Stan at 3 p.m. There was no visit from 1-3 p.m. at the hospital and I couldn't bear the thought of not being there when he left.

The nurse looked at me and said, "I know this is conflicting with visiting hours ending before he leaves but I am going to speak to the doctors for you, okay? See if somehow you can stay," he said reassuringly.

I started seeing God's favor firsthand. Just before 1 p.m. the nurse once again came into the room and started closing all the blinds of the windows facing the hallway as well as the doors.

At the same time, a hospital announcement was heard over the speaker system, "Visiting hours are now over and we ask all visitors to please leave the hospital."

The nurse looked at me knowing I heard the announcement and said, "Oh they just said something, I couldn't hear what it was," and smiled at me.

Stan started laughing and it took me a couple of seconds to realize what was happening.

The nurse had spoken to the doctor and he permitted me to stay until Stan was collected by the air team. I could breathe for another few hours and spend as much time as possible with Stan.

We kept watching the helipad as time grew closer. We did not expect to hear what the nurse walked in and announced.

"Wow, Mr. Gregory, you are flying first class to WMC. The team has just arrived by ambulance. They will transport you to the airport ten minutes away where the medical jet is waiting," he announced.

"WHAT? A JET?" I said loudly. "Yes ma'am, your husband is flying in style. The ambulance is at the ED and the staff is on their way up as we speak," he said with great excitement.

I couldn't believe what I was hearing. This was God's hand.

Within minutes, two flight nurses and an ambulance driver walked into the room introducing themselves. They had bags over their shoulders and a thin gurney piled with more equipment and gear.

Dressed in very cool flight suits and looking very professional, it felt like the rescue team had arrived.

"Good afternoon, Mr. Gregory. We are so sorry we are late but we are here to transport you to Westchester Medical Center. I am Flight Nurse Kelly and this is Flight Nurse Josh.

We will be preparing you for the flight. It will take quite some time but we will get you to the airport as soon as possible." Kelly explained and looked over at me.

"Are you his wife?" she asked.

"Yes, I am. Liesl. Thank you SO much for helping him," I said.

She smiled at me and said, "It is our pleasure. Please give me your mobile number. I will call you later tonight as soon as we have him settled in at WMC?"

"Thank you so much. Absolutely," I said as I started writing my name and number on her file with the pen she handed me.

They started unpacking all their equipment as Stan had to be transferred onto their equipment and off of Rochester General's. The process commenced by transferring one IV line at a time while they kept asking the nurse medical questions about Stan's history and current condition.

It felt like I was watching a movie, like I was being separated from being *in* the movie to only watching it. I wanted to press pause and catch my breath.

There was a sense of excitement in the room but reality kept setting in for me. The staff would make small talk and I made sure I was out of the way while they were moving around the bed constantly.

A sudden sadness came over me. It was as if I was removed from my body and watching things in slow motion. This was possibly the last time I would see my husband alive and instantly tears started flowing.

I stepped out of the room trying not to let Stan see me breaking down and walked into a corner in the hallway just outside his room. A nurse walked by and noticed I was crying.

She had so much compassion in her eyes as she walked over to me.

"Are you ok?" she asked and offered a folded tissue out of her pocket while putting her arm on my shoulder.

"Reality is tough to face," I uttered and she saw I was close to sobbing.

She stretched her arms out to me and offered a hug. At that moment, I didn't think about anything except I needed comfort in this stranger's arms. I needed a shoulder and I took her up on the offer and walked into her open arms.

After a few seconds, I stepped back and took a big breath trying to compose myself.
"Thank you, I will be back in there in a minute," I said to the nurse.

"You take all the time you need, okay?" she reassured and walked back into Stan's room.

I took a few more deep breaths, wiped my eyes, and took my place back in the room behind all the staff. I made sure Stan could see I was there but standing back so the crew could do their job.

Flight Nurse Josh was busy asking a staff member about the Impella readings.

They were going to take their machine and bring it back to Rochester on a later flight that evening as they didn't have one on board.

Before the flight crew had even arrived, the nurse had offered Stan some Oxycodone for the pain. He accepted as his chest hurt from the Impella insertion spot and he knew he was going to be moving a lot with the flight and ambulance drive.

We laughed when the flight nurse asked the hospital nurse to pass his oxygen line so she could put it onto their oxygen tank.

Excitedly, Stan said, "Oh, I don't need that!"
The flight nurse looked at him confused thinking there is no way a guy in his shape is not needing oxygen.

I started laughing and said, "I think that's the Oxycodone having an opinion on the oxygen right now".

"He had Oxy?" the nurse asked, looking at the hospital nurse.

"Yes, about 30 minutes ago, it's in his chart," and we started laughing.

"You need the oxy-gen, Mr. Gregory, but no more Oxycodone for you tonight, alright? You're getting your Oxy's confused," the nurse said and we all laughed again.

Just before five o'clock, they had Stan all wrapped up. Literally. He was wrapped up in a parachute-looking sleeping bag to help with his temperature control; safe in his traveling cocoon.

"You can follow us out of the ED if you like, Mrs. Gregory," the ambulance driver said.

"Thank you so much," I said and looked back at the staff seeing Stan off.
"Thank you so much for everything you did for Stan and I promise, when he has his new heart we will come and say hi to you all," I said trying to make sure they all know I am grateful to each of them.

"That is a deal!" the nurse said and a choir of "good lucks" and "all the bests" followed as we walked into the hallway heading to the ED.

As we walked out of the ambulance entrance double doors, Flight Nurse Kelly stopped and turned to me.

"You can say goodbye now as we will load him into the ambulance in a minute, it's a little cold outside," she said.

This was the moment I needed to be stronger than ever. I could not cry in front of Stan. I did not want him to think I thought he was not going to make it. I needed to be positive.

He was all cocooned and could not do much else but kiss me. I leaned over and kissed him.
"Bye handsome, I will see you on Monday. And you call me anytime, okay? Your phone and charger are in the bag the nurse has. Stay strong and I love you," I said and kissed him again quickly as I could feel the tears well up.

"I love you, too. I will call you when I can," Stan said as they pulled him closer to the ambulance.

"I will call you later tonight once he is settled at WMC. We will take good care of him," Nurse Kelly said.

"Thank you so much," I replied and turned to walk to the car.

I knew Stan could not see me and I also knew I was not going to be able to hold the tears back much longer.

I made it to the car and as I fell into the seat and sobbed. It felt like my world was crumbling and I didn't have any control over what was happening. I have always been someone who wanted to fix everything and this time it was out of my control.

It was dark outside and I needed to find the clinic across the road to do my COVID test. After I managed to get my composure back, I called Stewart. I needed him to feel updated, I could only imagine how he must have felt with Stan being his only sibling and being miles away.

I sat in the car park for a few more minutes and decided I was going to do the COVID test the next morning. I wanted to get home and relax. If I went the next morning I would also have an extra day before I needed to show a new test.

As I drove past the airport I looked over and wondered if Stan's jet had already taken off. A sense of loneliness hit me. I had a lot to do before I could leave Monday morning.

About two hours later while doing laundry, my phone rang. I didn't recognize the number.

"Hello?" I answered.

"Hi, Mrs. Gregory, this is Nurse Kelly. "Stan wants to say hi quickly. His voice is a little hoarse from the flight but he is doing well and settled in with the Cardiac team here at the hospital," she said.

Before I could thank her I heard Stan's hoarse voice. It shocked me at first. He didn't sound like that when I said goodbye but the flight must have taken a lot out of him.

"Hey, honey. I am safe and I'll speak to you tomorrow morning, okay? I am super tired and need something to drink before I can speak," Stan said.

"Ok good, let them take care of you and I will speak to you in the morning when you can." I said.

"I'll call you. I love you," Stan said before the nurse took the phone again.

"He did very well, Mrs. Gregory, and the hospital will be in contact tomorrow, okay?" Kelly said.

"Thank you, Kelly. I appreciate it," I said.

"You're welcome, sleep well," she said before she hung up.

Again I called Stewart and messaged all the family to let them know Stan made it safely. I was so tired. After a warm shower, some leftovers out of the fridge, and a cup of coffee I went to bed. I started praying as I lay there in the dark.

"Papa? Tonight I feel especially alone. I know You will never leave me or forsake me but Papa I feel so alone. I do not know why we have to go through this experience but You will have to hold my hand. I feel lost.

Please be with Stan. Please keep him safe and Papa please let me be able to see him Monday. NO, I take that back, THANK YOU for letting me see Stan on Monday and THANK YOU for keeping him safe.

You have taught me to pray in the positive and that is what I am going to do.

Papa, I know you have a plan. I cannot see that plan from my little perspective but I believe in You. I believe you are my Father and a Father wants only the best for their children.

Jesus I will step into 2 Corinthians 5:7, 'For I live by faith, not by sight.' Papa, I have no sight right now. I have no idea where this road is leading to but I know you are my healer, my provider, my Father. I know you want only the best for me and Stan.

Thank you for helping me over the next few days to get everything done that I need to do and thank you for reminding me of what I might forget. Thank you for you protection over Stan. In the name of Jesus Christ I command all that is not from You Papa, to leave Stan and his surroundings RIGHT NOW!

Thank you for sending your Angels to protect and watch over him.

Papa, help me sleep tonight. Help Stan sleep. Help his body to rest so that he has the strength to fight through this battle Jesus.

Papa, I know he loves you too. I know he is seeing you as the Great Man who lives in church but Papa I pray that you make Yourself known to him in a way he has never experienced. May he experience you as a friend, as a best friend, like I experience you. Not some Mighty Lord but a friend, someone he can speak to anywhere, any time, all the time, oh Papa, please, make this journey one that draws us both closer to you.

I love you Papa, I love you, thank you for…"

That was one of the many nights I fell asleep during prayer.

CHAPTER 2

God's Promise

Saturday, November 13, 2021

With organ donation there is a horrible false belief and false guilt that many patients awaiting organs feel. They feel a guilt that someone has to die for them to live. That is false. The death of the donor has nothing to do with the donor recipient.

The donor has an appointment date with God. Nothing can change that. The donor doesn't sacrifice their life to become a donor.

You become a donor the moment you have no more use for the body you have carried. A transplant miracle happens only after a tragedy happens. Not the other way around.

A tragedy was about to happen to a family we didn't know, while a miracle was busy unfolding for us.

I was up early making lists of chores I needed to do at the house and things I needed to pack. How do you pack for a trip when you don't have ANY idea how long you are going to be there? I reasoned that I could find a laundromat somewhere and was not going to pack too much unnecessarily.

I arranged for the car's wheel bearing to be fixed and for an oil change. The trip was a five to six hour drive and I needed a reliable vehicle in the unknown world I was about to enter.

First thing in the morning, I headed to Urgent Care for my COVID test. Thankfully with no waiting time and I was assured I would get my results by email the following day.

Shortly after, I called Stan and he sounded much better than the night before. This gave me renewed hope. We kept the conversation short with all I had to do in preparation to leave as well as the interruptions of the staff asking him questions.

In the afternoon, I was busy in the kitchen doing dishes, throwing out food that might go off while we were away, and listening, and singing along to worship music.

"Please Papa, please let Stan be ok," I prayed out loud and then something incredible happened.

Nothing short of a miracle.

I heard God say, in a voice so clear I remember it to this day. "***I am going to perform a miracle in Stan's life. Stan is going to be just fine, I am not done with him yet,***" God said.

Immediately I burst into tears, a flood of emotion cloaked me. Tears of relief quickly followed by an overwhelming sense of sadness. The sadness I felt was for the donor and the donor's family.

The realization that there will be a death of a donor. I sobbed in my kitchen that Saturday afternoon for this person and their family.

It felt like I was mourning this person's upcoming death. Someone I had never met, someone I will never get to meet here on earth.

It was the most peculiar, most incredible experience and I held onto God's words, "*I am going to perform a miracle in Stan's life. Stan is going to be fine, I am not done with him yet.*"

I prayed for this donor's soul. For their family and the tragedy that they were about to experience. An appointment with God, most possibly not expected at the time.

It was an incredible relief I felt for Stan and there my focus would lie. I continued praising God, singing in the kitchen, and repeating His words to myself over and over.

We were about to go on a journey of blind faith, but I KNEW God and trusted His plan.

By the evening I had accomplished what I set out to, including the car all set for travel. I made sure I had enough cash on me for the trip. It was time to find a place to stay down in the big city.

I was speaking to a friend who knows more about the city than I and she suddenly stopped during our conversation and said she would call me back in a bit.

I assumed she had something pop up on her side that needed her immediate attention. I continued searching for hotels and other accommodations close to the hospital.

My friend called me back after a couple of minutes and said she called a business associate of their company who lives in NYC and this friend was going to book a hotel for me for a week. I was blown away by God's favor and the goodness from a complete stranger.

Thank you, Lord! Within minutes, I was all set with a place to stay for a week. A fancy hotel only ten minutes from the hospital. God was showing favor through perfect strangers during such an unknown time.

My friend then blessed me even more by sending me a gift voucher to buy groceries down in the city. God is so good!

He was already showing me He is taking care of EVERY detail and He will continue to be our provider especially during this time.

Around 9 pm my phone rang. It was Stan.

"Hey you! What's up? How are you feeling?" I answered.

"Hey, honey. They are moving me to the Medical ICU from the Cardiac ICU as I have tested positive for COVID," Stan said and my heart sank.

"Here, speak to the nurse," Stan said and a nurse continued to introduce herself to me.

"Hi, Mrs. Gregory, we are just about to move your husband. His COVID test came back positive so he needs to go to isolation for fourteen days but we will take good care of him. Are you coming down on Monday?" she asked.

"Yes, oh my word, is he okay? Will I be able to see him?" I asked and she assured me as long as I have a negative PCR test result I will be able to see him.

Stan's voice took over the line again, "Honey, I am fine. I will call you tomorrow morning or later tonight depending on if I get to sleep, okay? I love you," Stan said.

"I love you too, please keep me updated," I said.

"I will honey, bye," Stan replied.

Stan didn't want me to worry but I knew him all too well and he was also trying to reassure himself by telling me he was doing fine. I would always be the reassuring one in the relationship but somehow he felt he needed to be strong for me too during this time where I was not able to see him.

I was petrified that I would take the trip down and not be able to see Stan. Would COVID end up causing his death as he is so weak already? Will this delay the evaluation process for two weeks?

I quickly became aware of the enemy trying to control my thoughts and immediately shifted my focus.

I had to keep going and have faith! I needed to believe in the promise of God. "***I am going to perform a miracle in Stan's life.***"

I fell asleep with a sense of peace amongst the signs of doom surrounding us. God's got our backs. But the roller coaster ride was far from over.

Sunday, November 14, 2021

Another early morning, making sure I was able to tick off everything on my list. A good friend of Stan, Mark Fox, called and asked if he could drop off a little travel basket his wife, Amy, had put together for me. He stopped by and dropped the nicest little basket of goodies for me.

So thoughtful, from microwave popcorn for the hotel, energy bars, gum, tissues, drinks, a gift card and so much more including a book to read. The kindness and support of family and friends gave me such a sense of calm. I realized I was not alone. I didn't have to face this challenge by myself. I had the support of incredible people. I was surrounded by love.

I gave Mark a house key as he offered to water plants and check in on everything every once in a while. He wouldn't be the last with something to offer.

This same day, one day before I left on my journey to meet up with Stan, God overflowed us with His goodness. So many friends dropped off small gifts and donations. The goodness of God was overwhelming.

I kept checking my email for my COVID test results. I was worried with Stan testing positive that I may be positive too. The enemy relished in messing with my mind.

Thank God the result was negative and I now had my paperwork in place to see Stan on Monday.

I called Stan before bed and briefly spoke to him as he sounded tired. I reassured him that God is not done with him and even though his level of faith might not have been where I was, he wanted to believe in this miracle God promised more than anything.

Later in the afternoon my daughter, Zaan Austen, called me to give me an update on Stan. She and her husband, Taylor, were on a mission trip to New Jersey and they stopped to visit Stan on the way back home.

Zaan knew I was worried and she tried to only share the good news but she, weeks later, told me she was extremely worried. The nurse told her we should not get our hopes up too soon.

I am still saddened that a nurse had to give her personal opinion to my daughter and almost make her lose hope. This nurse didn't know my God and she didn't know the promise He gave to perform a miracle in Stan's life.

By evening I was ready, all packed. All locked up. All security cameras in place. The house was ready for winter or however long we would be gone.

I had a warm shower, and light dinner and tried to get to bed early after I gave Stan another quick call. He sounded tired again but I understood he was very ill so I could not expect an energetic response during our conversations.

I assured him I would leave at 8 am the next morning which would give me plenty of time to find everything and be there for visiting hours in the afternoon.

It was lights out early for me to get enough rest. I was about to embark on an incredible journey.

CHAPTER 3

Blind Faith

Monday, November 15, 2021 – Stan's 65 birthday

At 2 a.m. my phone rang. It was Stan. This cannot be good.

"Stan?" I answered.

"Honey, I can't breathe," I heard Stan's muffled voice.

I could hear the nurse walk into the room and argue with him about taking the oxygen mask off his face.

"You got to keep this on Mr. Gregory, you are very sick and you need this right now, please," I heard her say.

She didn't realize Stan was on the phone with me. I kept quiet trying to listen to what was happening. I was terrified. I didn't want to let her know I was there because she might say Stan shouldn't be on the phone. I kept quiet and continued listening.

I heard her leave the room and heard Stan's voice faint, "Liesl, I can't breathe."

I could hear the panic in his voice. The heart monitor was going crazy in the background. Stan had struggled with breathing before so I knew it was not due to COVID but that he was panicking. I had to remain calm.

"Stan, listen to my voice, okay? Do not speak, just listen. You are ok, you are going to be ok. Just take a few deep breaths. As deep as you can," I coached him in the calmest, clearest voice I could muster.

I heard him trying to follow my instructions.

"That's it, honey. Keep breathing. Slowly, deeply, in through your nose, out through your mouth. There you go. Keep doing that. Smell the roses, blow out the candles. You are okay!" I kept saying.

I could hear the heart monitor slow down as he took control of his breathing and his heartbeat slowed down.

"Do you want me to pray for you?" I asked and I could hear him saying faintly, "Yes."

"Ok, you keep your eyes closed. Keep breathing like you are doing. No speaking. I will pray, okay?" I said.

I started praying out loud for Stan. Reminding Stan about the promise of God. The longer I prayed the more I could hear him calm down.

"Papa, I know you didn't bring me all the way into Stan's life for this to end here. Thank you for just calming him right now Jesus. Allow Stan to breathe deeper and help him feel the air going into his lungs," I prayed.

"Breathe as deep as you can honey, God is with you. Just believe. You are not alone," I told Stan.

"Papa, thank you for filling Stan's room with a feeling of peace that he has never experienced before. A calm that is only from You Papa. Clear Stan's lungs so he can breathe, deeper and deeper," I continued praying.

My prayer was combined with instruction for Stan.

I prayed for about an hour and around 3 a.m. I said, "Honey I am going to hang up and get ready to leave. I am going to leave right now and I will be right outside the hospital, ok?"

I felt that maybe being closer to him physically might also make him feel more reassured that he is not alone.

He mumbled "ok" and I hung up.

Stan did *not* sound good and at that moment the enemy used doubt to make me wonder if Stan would make it through the night. My battle between faith and doubt was only starting.

I managed to get ready quickly and left a few minutes later. The darkness surrounded me in the early hours of the morning. Blindly following a GPS to the destination, Westchester Medical Center, New York.

A few bags of things I thought I might need while away stacked in the back of the car. The roads were quiet.

I prayed for most of the trip. About two hours into the journey I heard the car making a noise again. The enemy was desperate to make me lose faith and make me panic. I kept praying that God would get me to the city safely.

The first few hours of the trip, I allowed myself to forget God's promise. I allowed the enemy into my mind. Hearing the panic in Stan's voice early that morning made me believe that maybe that could have been our last conversation. I did not think Stan was going to make it through the night.

Around 7:30 a.m. my phone rang. It was Stan.

"Stan?" I answered quickly.

I was shocked yet pleasantly surprised at the voice I heard. Stan sounded like the old chirpy Stan I knew. NOTHING like the man who called me at 2 a.m.

"Hi honey, where are you at?" he asked like the 2 am conversation never happened.

"Hey!! Oh my word, it is so good to hear you sounding better. I am about an hour out of the city according to the GPS, going to hit Monday morning traffic, I guess. How are you feeling?" I asked.

"Okay. I just couldn't breathe last night with that mask on my face," Stan replied.

"Hey! Happy birthday, old man," I said.

Stan laughed, "I am four now."

Stan would always laugh when he did something silly and say, "I am three, almost four."

"I can't wait to see you. I am going to hang up and call you when I reach the hospital, okay? Traffic is getting heavier. I can't check into the hotel till 3 p.m. so I am just going to hang in the parking lot or see if I can get a coffee at the hospital," I explained.

"Sounds good, honey. Let me know. I love you," Stan said.

"I love you too, see you in a bit," I said and hung up.

It was a great relief to hear Stan's voice and to hear liveliness in him. Sunrise seemed to bring him out of the nighttime anxiety.

I called Stewart to give him an update and then set my focus on the last section of the journey.

I arrived at the hospital and found a spot in the car park right in front of the hospital's main entrance. I had all my paperwork printed to be able to see Stan.

Our marriage certificate as my driver's license was still in my maiden name, my negative COVID PCR test, and anything else they could need from me. I was prepared and nothing was going to stop me from seeing my husband.

Ready to roll with hours to spare.

I made good use of the time and made a few needed calls. I called the hospital general inquiries to ask where I could have a COVID test done while down in the city.

Yet another blessing. There was a tent set up right next to the hospital with drive-through testing by appointment.

They gave me the number to call for bookings and I managed to get an appointment for the next day which would hopefully give me a result by Thursday when I would need a new result. This math was too much for my emotionally wrecked mind.

This was going to be my routine for a while. I chose the simple way and booked a PCR test for every Tuesday and every Friday for two weeks in advance. Then after two weeks, same thing.

I would have testing done daily if it meant I could continue to see Stan.

At 1:30 p.m. I went into the hospital lobby and asked if I had everything they needed for me to see my husband. They confirmed I was all set.

What a relief. I could take a deep breath and realized I would forcefully have to breathe deeper as my breathing became shallow over the past few days feeling so stressed.

I was checked in by the front desk and told I would be given an access sticker at 2 p.m. when visiting hours start. Someone would be reading out the names and visitors could step forward to collect their access sticker.

Soon there was a long line of people checking in. I was just in time to miss the crowd and knew I would need to be there at least 30 minutes before visiting hours each day to avoid the rush.

I was learning all the tricks which would make my life easier over the next few days, weeks, months, and years… I had no clue how long this journey would be.

At 2 p.m. a small crowd gathered at the elevator lobby. This would be a daily occurrence. Everyone would wait for their names to be read and then collect their access sticker to visit their loved ones.

I caught the eye of two ladies, a mom, and a daughter and we shared a smile.

Finally, my name was read. I collected my sticker and walked up to the elevators. My destination was the 2nd-floor Medical ICU also known as the MICU.

While in the elevator I received a phone call. It was not a contact on my phone but I recognized the area code as one from the Westchester Hospital area.

"Hello?" I answered.

A female voice introduced herself but I missed the name due to the bad connection in the elevator.

"Mrs. Gregory, where are you at the moment?" the lady asked.

"I am in the elevator on the way to see my husband, why?" I said.

"Oh no. You won't be able to see him," the voice said.

My heart sank. After ALL this I was NOT going to be able to see Stan? The voice continued, "He is not in the room. He is in the OR." the voice said.

"WHAT? For what? Why is he in surgery?" I asked frantically.

"He is having a procedure done," she said.

The elevator doors opened and I felt I could breathe again.

"I have not been notified he needs a procedure- What procedure?" I demanded an answer.

I noticed the sign to turn right to the MICU and I was now on a mission to get to Stan. I needed answers and felt I could only get those answers by speaking to someone face to face.

"Look, I am not sure who you are but I suggest you come to his room right now and meet me there so we can clear this up," I said in a short and almost rude tone and hung up.

Taken aback and confused by this news I started walking even faster to get to Stan.

When I reached the MICU entrance I rang the bell on the intercom. A couple of seconds later a friendly female voice answered.

"I am here to see my husband Stan Gregory," I said hoping not to have a response that I was not able to see him.

"Come in," the voice said.

The doors opened and I walked to the front desk. A friendly face welcomed me.

"Good afternoon, Mrs. Gregory, I am happy to see you had a safe trip down." she said with a smile.

"Thank you so much. Can you tell me, is my husband in the OR," I asked with urgency.

She looked at me confused and said, "No, he is in his room at the end of the hallway to the right."

She shrugged off the confusion and continued explaining, "Nurse Andrew is with him and will give you an update. Why did you think he was in the OR?" she asked with a renewed look of confusion.

"I just had a call from someone who said he was in the OR. I missed the person's name as there was bad reception in the elevator. As long as he is ok." I said.

"I have no idea who would have called you, that's strange. He is definitely in his room. Please put on this gown, and you have to double mask and then place this face shield on too. Oh and a very fashionable hair net. The nurse will give you a set of gloves. Welcome, Mrs. Gregory," she said and handed me a whole pack of items with a smile.

"Thank you so much," I replied and started walking down the hallway with my kit in hand.

I walked faster as I now needed to see Stan with my own eyes to feel assured he is ok.

As I approached the end of the hallway the nurse got up from his seat and greeted me, "Hi, you must be Mrs. Gregory?"

He was sitting in his little workstation at the end of the hallway outside Stan's room. There were glass walls to the room with glass double doors.

"Hi Andrew. Yes I am. How is Stan?" I asked and could see Stan through the glass wall.

I immediately felt relief knowing he was not in an OR and was awake and in his room. I wondered what purpose that elevator call had in this situation. Had I not endured enough?

He was staring at the television but saw movement and looked towards the glass. When he saw me, he smiled. At that moment it was like a mountain was lifted off me.

I could not gear up fast enough. Andrew helped me to make sure everything was fitted correctly.

Gown, double mask, face shield, hair net, and gloves. I was instructed that when I leave the room the items needed to be removed and placed in separate bins at the door.

While putting on the gown I asked, "How is he doing, Andrew?"

"He is stable this morning. He had a bit of a panic attack during the night but I spoke to the doctor about possible medication to help him if it happens again. This is a lot to take in," Andrew assured me.

"Yes, he called me when he was panicking and I just calmed him as best I could. Would the doctors be around this afternoon so I could have a word with them?" I asked.

"For sure, they are in and out all the time," Andrew said.

At last, I was able to walk into the room. Stan was laying down at no more than a 30 degree upright position due to the heart pump which had access through his groin.

His lunch was still on the tray next to him.

"Hey handsome, you look older today. Happy birthday!!" I said.

Stan smiled and said, "Yeah, ok."

He has never been one to make a big deal out of a birthday. Stan told me how different things are at this hospital and how he panicked during the night. I assured him I would be with him from 2-6 p.m. every day while he was in the hospital.

I could only imagine what he was going through. This journey was tough on me but it was very tough on Stan in a completely different way.

Stan was physically struggling, as well as emotionally. His weak heart caused him to sleep through most of the process making him completely unaware of the details. He was poked and prodded all day long but the toll of being his advocate was also taking a toll on me.

I was living the details. Answering the questions. Finding the medical history they requested, making the phone calls to doctors to find past visit dates, and results. I saw the reality of the situation more clearly and my mental and emotional stress was reaching a level I have never experienced before.

Later when Stan dozed off, I had time to scan the room. It was a big room with a large window. There was a view of the car park in front of the hospital.

In the corner was a large and very noisy HEPA filter, a television mounted on the wall, and right next to it a camera and intercom. The camera allowed the nurses to watch the patients closely even from different rooms.

There was a whiteboard under the TV which read:

Patient: Stan Gregory
Doctor: Dr. Lanier
Date: 11/15/2021
Nurse: Andrew

Stan had so many IV lines going into his center line in his neck. The Impella pump next to the bed, still working hard at supporting Stan's failing heart.

Stan had a different colored gown from the one he wore at the hospital in Rochester. His nose was a little red from the irritation of the oxygen tube. The bedsheet was pulled up over his arms.

I pulled up a chair as close as I could without bumping into any equipment and sat down slowly. I reached under the sheet to find Stan's hand, trying not to wake him. I needed to feel his touch.

A doctor walked into the room and introduced himself to me. Stan did not wake up.

"Good afternoon, I am Doctor Lanier, you must be Mrs. Gregory?" he asked.

"Hi Doctor, yes. How is he doing?" I asked.

He took a step back drawing me away from Stan like he wanted to speak in private and make sure Stan didn't hear us. Stan was still sleeping. I slowly stood up and stepped over, closer to the doctor.

"Mrs. Gregory, your husband is very ill and we are doing everything we can to get him onto the transplant list but if he doesn't qualify then I am afraid we will have to transfer him to hospice," he said.

I had never experienced a gut punch in my life but this was a gut and face punch at the same time.

I knew Stan was ill but I guess a level of denial didn't allow me to believe he was THIS ill. To hear the words that he is busy dying was a reality punch in the gut.

"How long does the evaluation take?" I asked.

"We are doing things as quickly as possible and will keep you up to date. We have your number to call you if you are not here and please feel free to ask the nurse to call us if you have any questions, we are always around," he said.

I had so many questions I wanted to ask but the shock to hear my husband might have to go to hospice to die still had me completely paralyzed.

"Thank you doctor," I said and he left the room.

I fell back into the chair. Sadness threatened to overwhelm me but I grabbed onto the promise of God once more. "***I am going to perform a miracle in Stan's life. I am not done with him yet.***" I clung onto those words.

I was not going to allow the enemy free space in my mind again. I softly started singing a worship song, over and over, "I will worship while I wait for our miracle. I will worship for the both of us":

While I Wait

Lincoln Brewster

Deep within my heart, I know You've won
I know You've overcome
And even in the dark, when I'm undone
I still believe it

I live by faith, and not by sight
Sometimes miracles take time

While I wait, I will worship
Lord, I'll worship Your name
While I wait, I will trust You
Lord, I'll trust You all the same

When I fall apart, You are my strength
Help me not forget
Seeing every scar, You make me whole
You're my healer

I live by faith, and not by sight
Sometimes miracles take time
I live by faith, and not by sight
Sometimes miracles take time

While I wait, I will worship
Lord, I'll worship Your name

While I wait, I will trust You
Lord, I'll trust You all the same

You're faithful every day
Your promises remain
You're faithful every day
Your promises remain
You're faithful every day
Your promises remain
You're faithful every day
Your promises remain

Though I don't understand it
I will worship with my pain
You are God, You are worthy
You are with me all the way

So while I wait, I will worship
Lord, I'll worship Your name
Though I don't have all the answers
Still I trust You all the same

Tears streamed down my cheeks. I FELT God at that moment. The Holy Spirit was present in that room. I BELIEVED that He was going to perform a miracle. The tough part was accepting that sometimes miracles take time and sometimes things have to get much worse before we can recognize the miracle.

I had no idea how dark things were going to become over the next few days. The rollercoaster was about to reach full speed.

Different doctors and nurses came in and out of the room all the time. All checking different things as part of the evaluation. Later in the afternoon, another doctor walked in with two younger doctors behind him.

"Good afternoon, I am Dr. Levine. I am one of the doctors helping to get your husband onto the list," he said.

I had no idea at that moment what a role this doctor was going to play in Stan's future. Dr. Avi Levine.

"Hi, doctor, nice to meet you. Thank you so much", I said. "I have a few questions for you if you have time?" I said and he stepped closer.

"Of course, what would you like to know?" he said.

I could see in his body language he was sincerely wanting to reassure me with whatever I wanted to know. Stan once again dozed off, he simply couldn't stay awake.

"What are my husband's chances of getting onto the list? I mean, he is 65 today. Is that not too old?" I asked.

"Oh no, not at all! We have done transplants on patients much older than him. His age is not so much the deciding factor," he explained.

"So what makes him qualify?" I asked.

"Well, there are many things we look at. His health, other than the heart condition. Your husband is not diabetic and doesn't have any other health issues. He is not a smoker. Does he use alcohol?" he asked.

"No, he used to have a drink every once in a while but recently he has not had any alcohol," I replied.

"That's another big plus. And we look at many other aspects. Does he use recreational drugs? Does he have emotional support? Does his support have support? What is his mental health like? We will have the social worker and the transplant psychologist also speak to you both. Right now things look positive to have him listed. We just need to complete all the testing and have all the work completed but I am positive at this stage he will make the list," he said.

I wanted to start crying and hug him. I needed this breath of hope. This was one of the many moments where Dr. Levine would bring calmness to the situation. I felt like I could breathe again.

I sighed in relief and I might have even grabbed at my heart in relief.

"We are doing everything we can, okay?" he reassured.

"Thank you, doctor. Thank you," I replied.

"It's a pleasure. Be prepared for many questions from various people over the next couple of days. It's all part of the information we need. Feel free to ask any questions," he said and I could see a smile in his eyes.

A very reassuring smile. I might have also spotted wings and a halo in that moment.

"Oh, doctor, what about the COVID? Do you think he has COVID because I have not seen any symptoms since I arrived earlier?" I asked.

"Look, we are not sure. He doesn't show many symptoms but it was a positive result so we need to have him isolated. Rest assured this does not stop the evaluation process. We are continuing anyway," he said.

Once again, music to my ears.

"Thank you, doctor. I appreciate what you are doing. Thank you," I said.

"It's our pleasure," he said.

He asked the nurse about some readings on Stan's Impella and seemed pleased with the answer.

"We will see you later ok? Hang in there," he said as he left the room.

"Thank you doctor," I replied.

If I was asked to describe an Angel at that time, Dr. Levine would have been it.

The rest of the afternoon was spent caring for Stan. Helping him with eating and drinking because laying down doing the simplest things was a challenge. The last thing we needed was for him to choke on his food.

Nurse Andrew sat right outside his room watching him on his monitor and checking on him through the glass window in the hallway. Every once in a while he would gear up and come into the room to change an IV or check the pump readings.

I felt reassured Stan was in good hands. I needed to see this for myself, to KNOW they are doing whatever they can. The unknown became more known, even though the future was still a mystery and in God's hands.

I could see yet another person starting to gear up in the hallway. She walked in and introduced herself as the transplant psychologist. I recognized her voice from the phone call earlier and before I could say anything she apologized for the misunderstanding.

I was relieved it was simply a misunderstanding rather than Stan being in the OR for something I didn't know about.

We spoke for a while and she asked if she could call me the following morning to ask a few questions for the evaluation.

"Of course!" I said.

I would do anything to help.

"Wonderful. It is easier to understand each other over the phone than through the double mask and face shield," she grinned.

"Absolutely! And you have my number," I said with a giggle.

"Yes, I do," she laughed. "My apologies again," she said.

"All in the past, we look forward now," I said and she confirmed with a big nod.

That evening I said goodbye to Stan and left for the hotel. I pulled the masks off walking out of the hospital main entrance. Breathing fresh, cold air was wonderful. I could take a few deep breaths of relief and breathed in new hope.

The hotel was beautiful and walking into my hotel room I felt like a spoiled child of Jesus. It was my little haven for the next seven days.

As had become the routine, I called Stewart and the kids with the day's updates. I decided to create a chat group where I could give updates to friends on a daily basis rather than have everyone ask and me trying to keep up with what I shared with them.

During times like this your world becomes so complicated that you have to do what you can to keep things simple.

I had a light meal, a shower, and watched some television while the day's events flashed through my mind.

Around 9 p.m. Stan called.

"Hey honey, will you pray for me again? It helped last night." he said.

This is not something Stan ever asked for and I could sense he was nervous about the night and possibly having another anxiety attack.

"Of course, I will!" I said and started praying.

We spoke for a little while and said goodnight. I had a strange sense of calm even in the chaos at that moment.

Tuesday, November 16, 2021

I woke up around early and opened the curtain to see what it looked like outside. I arrived the previous evening when it was dark outside. It was not quite light yet and I could only see a small part of the car park lit up with lights and trees in the distance. I made a cup of coffee.

Stan called shortly after and said he had a better night. He needed reassurance. I was going to be there for visiting hours later in the day and in the coming days, he would ask for this reassurance often.

It reminded me that the journey is not just tough on me but also for him. Very different angles of the same experience.

The morning was spent on the phone with the psychologist asking me about Stan's mental health and history. We got along well and she assured me she sees no issues from her side to approve Stan for the list.

After speaking to the social worker for more than an hour I came to realize how important it was for the transplant recipient to have a support system and for me, his first support, to also have support. It was one of the qualifying factors when deciding to list a patient. This made it clear that there was a long journey ahead. A tough one.

The social worker, Bryan, also called me and we spoke for quite some time. It became clearer that a big qualifying factor to be listed for transplant was if the patient had a strong support system.

In simple terms, they needed to know a transplant recipient was going to be supported and strong enough to first make it through surgery, but also to have a strong chance at a good quality of life in the future.

There were other little details I also learned. The patient should not have any broken skin, cuts, or scratches for example as the immune system is very weak after the transplant.

The immune system is suppressed with medication to ensure the body does not reject the new organ as a foreign body. Stan would be on these suppressants for the remainder of his life, if he received a donor heart.

My morning blessing was my dear friend Kim who called to say she started a go-fund-me account as she knew Stan is now not able to work and neither was I.

We also didn't know how long I would be in the city and bills kept coming. What a blessing our friends were and even total strangers who supported us.

Kim kept reassuring me I would be fine if anything happened to Stan. I then reassured her, explaining to her what happened in the kitchen that Saturday and that God was not done with him yet.

Kim kept trying to reassure me that IF anything happened and Stan didn't make it, I would be fine. But I wouldn't hear it.

I would keep saying, "He is going to be just fine, Kim!"

I felt God's favor and blessing every step of the way. Shortly before lunch I left for the hospital to make sure I got there before the long line of people wanting to check in to visit their loved ones.

As I sat waiting for 2 p.m. to arrive, I again noticed the mom and daughter from the day before. I walked to the local coffee shop to get a coffee and browsed around a little to familiarize myself with what might be 'home' for a while.

When I reached the MICU entrance I was greeted by the now almost familiar mom and her daughter. They had just rung the bell on the intercom.

"I hope we don't have to wait as long as we had to yesterday," the mom said with a slight laugh.

"Did you wait long?" I asked and the mom and daughter both said, "Oh yes."

"Frustrating when you want to get to your loved one to spend every minute, right? A few minutes feels like an eternity," I replied.

"Absolutely," the daughter replied.

"Do you have a friend or family member here?" I asked.

The mom pointed to her daughter and said, "Her boyfriend is here."

"How about you?" the daughter asked.

"My husband," I replied.

The doors opened unexpectedly with no communications over the intercom.

"Well, all the best," I said as we walked in.

"You too," they both said and we walked our separate ways.

As I geared up, Stan noticed me through the glass and looked at the clock and tapped on his wrist, signaling I was late. His humor was still shining even though he was faced with so many challenges.

I walked in and his first words were, "You are late."

"Well, take that up with the front desk, why don't you, I was waiting for them to respond to the bell at the MICU entrance, okay?" I said and we both laughed.

Stan hadn't eaten much of his lunch yet and I started cutting up his chicken into bite-size pieces. It was hard enough to even see what was on the plate laying down, never mind trying to cut the food.

It made me feel like there was something I could help with so I made it my duty to come and feed him his lunch at 2 p.m. every day and then his dinner at 5:30 p.m., just before I would leave at 6 p.m. after visiting hours.

As usual, the afternoon was filled with doctors and nurses moving in and out of the room. A transplant team member asked if they could ask me a few questions outside. Stan fell asleep and they needed me to sign a few things as I was his medical proxy.

They spoke to me about signing up for what is called an 'at risk heart'. This would improve Stan's chances of receiving a heart quicker once he is listed.

An 'At risk heart' is a heart from a donor who might have struggled with addiction and possibly contracted Hepatitis through needle use.

The liver specialist explained to me that if the donor was Hepatitis positive they would immediately start Stan on treatment and most patients have no issues after treatment is completed.

Beggars can't be choosers and Stan was in a desperate situation. If this would increase his chances of survival, of getting a heart sooner, there was not much of a choice. I agreed to sign for an 'at-risk heart' option as well.

I was also given an option to list with another hospital but I felt that the care Stan was getting was what he needed and I was extremely happy with the care he got so I declined. I felt this is where God wanted us.

I called Stewart after the staff left as I needed confirmation I made the right decision and Stew was also a proxy for Stan.

"Absolutely. He cannot pick and choose right now," Stewart replied and I felt relieved that he agreed I did the right thing by signing up.

Being your loved one's proxy is a tough position when it comes to these decisions, but for us, Stan's survival was now a priority. Everything else could be dealt with later.

Visiting hours seemed to fly by and by the end of the visit I told Stan he was going to be just fine.

"I hope so," he said with a concerned look in his eyes.

"I KNOW so. You know what God told me in the kitchen on Saturday?" I said.

Stan had a curious look on his face, "What?" he asked.

"He is going to perform a miracle in your life and He is not done with you, Stanley Gregory!" I said as I cupped my hands over his cheeks looking into his eyes.

I could see tears well up in Stan's eyes.

"God's got you honey!" I said.

I left the hospital again around 6 p.m. and grabbed dinner on the way to the hotel. The routine of coming and going never felt frustrating to me. I was grateful to be able to be at Stan's side supporting him through this journey. I also made a promise, to him, and God, for better and worse.

The evening was spent relaxing, updating family and friends, and getting some much-needed rest. Just before I fell asleep I did my evening prayer with Stan over the phone again.

It was hard to believe what we had been through. It was only a week since I dropped Stan off at Rochester General Hospital ED.

This was just the beginning of the roller coaster. We were about to hit the high peak, the climax, and that long steep drop. The part where most close their eyes and just scream.

CHAPTER 4

Setbacks & Blessings

Wednesday, November 17, 2021

I was at the hospital early to check in. The mom and daughter team were checking-in early too. They came and stood next to me.

"How is your husband doing?" the mom asked.

"He is stable. He needs a heart transplant and they are busy with the evaluation to see if he will make the list but he is in the MICU because he tested positive for COVID the night after he was flown in from Rochester," I explained.

"Oh, my word," the mom said.

"My boyfriend was also flown in about a week ago with bad COVID symptoms. He has other health issues too but the other hospital was about to give up on him," the daughter explained.

"Where are you from?" I asked.

"Waverley in New York," they both replied.

"That's like the next town from where my daughter lives in Spencer, what a small world," I said.

"Oh yea, that's like home to us," the mom laughed.

"I am Liesl Gregory, by the way," I said.

The mom responded, "I am Candy Wagner and this is my daughter Karen Wagner. Her boyfriend is Dave Maroney."

"My husband is Stan," I responded. "So where are you staying?" I asked.

"In a hotel about a mile away," they replied. "And you?" they asked.

"In a hotel about ten minutes away," I replied.

Our conversation was disturbed by our names being called to collect access stickers. We got into the same elevator and wished each other's loved ones the best and said we would probably see each other around the next few days.

To our surprise, the MICU doorbell was answered in record time and we went our separate ways to the different rooms.

"Hi, how is Stan today?" I asked the nurse as I walked up to her station.

"He has just been for a CT Scan. He just got back. I am sure the doctor will be in any minute," the nurse explained.

I just assumed the CT scan was all part of the evaluation testing and I was not prepared for what the doctor was going to share as he came walking down the hallway.

"Mrs. Gregory, I am glad I am catching you," Dr. Levine said as he started gearing up with me to go into Stan's room.

"Is there a problem, doctor?" I asked as I could see some concern in his eyes.

"We just did a CT scan on Stan and he has suffered a small stroke. There is a small brain bleed so we are going to keep an eye on it," he explained.

A brain bleed? A stroke? I could not believe, or rather, I didn't WANT to believe what I was hearing.

I was dumbstruck. "What??? Is he ok? Will this affect the evaluation?" I asked.

"He is fine! No, it won't affect our evaluation, not at all. Neurology is keeping a close eye on him and I am confident he will be fine," Dr. Levine said.

We walked into the room together. Stan was awake and Doctor Levine brought him up to date on the results of the scan. Stan almost had no response and didn't seem to fathom the seriousness of what was happening.

He seemed to be 'different' somehow. As an empath, I am extremely sensitive to people's energy and the vibe in a room when I walk in. Stan's energy was different.

He seemed a little confused and not quite himself. This was normal behavior after a brain bleed but I didn't fully comprehend how my husband had instantly changed.

Dr. Levine again reassured me that everything is going ahead and they are keeping a close eye on him.

After he left the room I pulled Stan's lunch tray closer and started to feed him his lunch. He was grumpy, moody, and there was a definite change in his behavior. By the afternoon his grumpiness turned into rudeness.

We would often sit holding hands but this day was upsettingly different.

I reached out to take his hand and he shook his arm away and said, "Don't do that."

It was hard for me, an empath, not to take it personally. It was also tough because Stan was a stranger to me all of a sudden.

I was just by his side while he would look at me and randomly say the strangest things.

"Mike has the best meatballs, let's go get some pizza," he said.

Mike was a good friend of Stan who owned a Pizza shop close to our home. Stan's favorites included meatballs, pizza, or chicken.

"Sure, in a little while," I replied.

I knew from working with people with dementia you have to climb into their world and not argue with them. Stan was acting like someone suffering from dementia so I had to adapt to his world.

A few minutes later Stan would say, "Do you want to go watch a ballgame this weekend?"

"Sure honey, let's see what the weather is like on the weekend though, okay?" I replied.

He spoke no sense most of the day. It was a scary time for me but I had to be strong and keep it together.

Things seemed to be getting worse, not better. The irony is, when you are listed for a transplant, it's got to get worse before it gets better. You do not reach the top of the list as a healthy person. You need to be sick or sicker to reach the top of the list.

The rest of the day was the same statements from Stan over and over and he was grumpy all day. Nothing I seemed to want to help with was right. He wouldn't let me touch him. My husband felt like a stranger. I felt alone.

By early evening I was mentally exhausted. Tearful. I had to get out of there. Stan was argumentative and my gentle little compassionate soul could not bear it any longer.

I felt guilty for leaving early but it seemed like Stan was not even aware of time and visiting hours or anything "real" happening around him.

As I walked out of the room nurse Mimi said, "You are leaving early today?"

"I have to Mimi, I am mentally exhausted. He has been arguing with me all day and speaking no sense whatsoever," I said as I felt tears welling up.

Mimi was the sweetest lady and just beamed with compassion.

She opened her arms and stepped closer to hug me and said in her beautiful Jamaican accent, "You go and take care of yourself. I will take care of your husband, okay?"

I shed a couple of tears on her shoulder and composed myself as I grabbed my bag.

"Thank you, Mimi," I said as I walked off still struggling to keep my tears under control.

By the time I reached the car, I felt safe to let my composure go and burst into tears. It was a challenging and unexpected day.

I wanted to get back to the hotel. Shower and get in bed so I could continue my crying and feel sorry for myself some more. I call these my red wine and tissue box moments. My very own little pity party and no-one is invited.

Stan did not call me that night. I was not surprised as he was so confused. Maybe I was even relieved in some way. I cried myself to sleep.

Thursday, November 18, 2021

I arrived at the hospital a little early as usual. Candy and Karen were also early and we decided to have a coffee together at the coffee shop. They shared more about Karen's boyfriend, Dave, and the run-up to how he ended up at Westchester.

Similarly, I shared about Stan and it was good to have someone to speak to in person. We enjoyed each other's company and they immediately seemed like my tribe, my kind of people.

I was bracing myself for how Stan would be, praying he was in a better mental state than the previous day.

When it hit 2 o'clock we headed to the elevator.

"Good afternoon, how is Stan today?" I asked the nurse walking up to his room.

"He was a little agitated but he is stable. I believe the doctor wants another CT scan today but he should be around shortly to confirm the plan of action," the nurse explained.

I geared up and braced myself for what I was possibly walking in on. There was no smile or greeting from Stan. My husband was still a stranger.

"Liesl, can you get this bedpan out from under me," were his first words.

"Hi honey, sure," I said and walked over to the opposite side of the bed away from all the equipment.

I was surprised he was using a bedpan. Since the day they put the balloon pump in he simply had to let go of the protective covers they had set under him and then the staff would clean him up.

Stan had a huge problem with this at first because it's one of the less dignifying things about the process.

It was explained to me by a nurse that firstly they didn't want to move Stan too much by trying to get the pan under him and secondly it could tear the skin when he has been laying down for a long time.

I lifted his leg slightly to see if I could see a bedpan but knew I was not going to find anything.

"There is no bedpan," I said.

"There is, Liesl," Stan said, annoyed.

I looked again and confirmed to him there was nothing.

"Liesl! There is a bedpan. Can you get it out, please?" Stan demanded again, very annoyed, raising his voice slightly.

I realized he was even more confused than the day before. A doctor walked in and introduced himself as a Neurologist.

"Mrs. Gregory, have you noticed any behavior changes in your husband recently?" he asked.

"Yes, I have since yesterday. He is very confused and agitated," I replied.

"That is quite normal after suffering a bleed in that part of the brain. The behavior will pass," he said.

It will pass! Those words were like music to my ears.

"We are going to have the Impella pump replaced with a balloon pump today as we believe the Impella might have contributed to the brain bleed due to the blood thinners. We will then do another CT Scan to see where we are at," he explained.

"Thank you. Doctor, does this affect his chances of being listed? I asked.

"No, the heart transplant team is proceeding and we will see where we are at with the bleed in the next few hours," he replied.

"Thank you so much," I said as the doctor got ready to leave the room.

Stan was just staring at the doctor blankly. He was a total stranger to me and completely oblivious to the fact that I was now his advocate fighting for him to be listed.

There's something terrifying about seeing the person you love turn into a stranger overnight. It gave me the most overwhelming sense of loneliness.

After the doctor left the room, Stan continued complaining about the bedpan.

I thought maybe I should change the way I handle this and said, "Ok honey let me get it out," and pulled the protective sheet cover like I was removing something from under him.

He didn't say a word and a few seconds later he replied, "Liesl, it is still there!"

I was at a lack of words.

Nurse Andrew walked in and I asked him, "Andrew does Stan have a bedpan under him right now?"

Andrew looked at me very confused and said, "No?"

He looked at Stan and said, "You are fine, there is no bedpan."

Somehow because Andrew said it Stan was happy to accept it and left it at that.

Andrew looked at me as he was checking the IV lines and said, almost to reassure me I was not the one losing my mind, "He has been a little confused today."

"A LITTLE? You think?" I replied and giggled.

Andrew nodded and for a guy who always acted very straight-faced and professional, slipped out a little laugh. He just brought a sense of calm to the room whenever he was there.

Later that afternoon a doctor came in to say they were going to take him to the OR to place a balloon pump and then remove the Impella.

They explained it would take an hour or so and suggested I go have some coffee and take a break. A MUCH needed break!

That is exactly what I needed. I sat in the coffee shop watching the doctors and nurses come and go getting coffee, snacks, meals, and drinks. There was a constant hustle and bustle as people came to refuel.

I noticed a note on the table. It was about a special on limitless coffee. You pay $12 a month and get limitless coffee. WHAT? That sounded like a great deal. Especially with my regular breaks from the bedpan sagas.

I was paying almost $3 every time for a coffee and immediately signed up through their app. I also signed up for their rewards program. At this stage every penny saved helped.

An hour and a half passed and I made my way back to Stan's room slowly.

"He just got back. Everything went well," Andrew said as I arrived. "I am also going in now just to check the balloon pump once more".

We geared up and went into the room. Stan was quiet.

"Hey. How are you feeling?" I asked.

"Ok," Stan replied and that was about the full conversation before he dozed off.

I went and sat in the wide windowsill. I would often sit there when he fell asleep and stare at ambulances coming and going, people walking in and out and autumn leaves blowing across the car park. It reminded me there was a world outside the crazy little space we found our lives to be in at the moment.

Funny how you feel separated from the rest of the world in a moment like that. The world continues and is completely unaware of what you are dealing with.

I looked over at Stan and it hit me again just how sick he was. That he will have to go to hospice if he doesn't get listed. Now he has a brain bleed. Lord! How much worse does it need to get?

I assumed this condition would not count in his favor to get listed. The enemy wanted to mess with my mind at that moment and I rebuked it.

"Lord I am holding onto your promise" I kept saying and the song "While I wait, I will worship you," popped into my mind once again. I sat on that windowsill, softly singing that song for hours.

Around 4 p.m. Dr. Levine entered the room. I was not ready to hear more bad news but he came bearing great news amidst a dark outlook.

"I have good news," Dr. Levine said.

"OH doctor, I need good news, please share," I responded.

His eyes started smiling again.

"Stan is officially listed. He is on the transplant list," he said.

I could hardly believe my ears. Tears welled up in my eyes.

"Thank you thank you thank," I kept shouting while keeping my hands in a prayer position on my chest. "So the brain bleed is okay?" I asked.

"Yes. Neurology has cleared him. The bleeding has stopped and they expect a full recovery from the bleed," Dr. Levine explained.

"Thank you, Doctor Levine. Thank you so, so much," I said and it felt like such an understatement for the emotion I was feeling.

I wanted to grab him and hug him in gratitude!

"You are so welcome. Now we wait for a heart to become available," Dr. Levine said.

"It will, I am sure. God is in control," I replied.

"Yes, he is," Dr. Levine said.

He looked over at Stan who just stared at him as he was still very confused about what was going on around him.

"We will see you in the morning, Stan," Dr. Levine said.

"Yes, thank you, Dr. Levine," Stan said very politely.

Almost as if he understood what was happening.

It was the biggest relief I felt in a long time and a huge ray of hope started shining through. This was nothing short of a miracle to me. I took a few deep breaths of relief.

Shortly after, Stan's dinner arrived. I cut up his meal and fed him, just too happy to see that he was still eating, even if it was a little.

After visiting hours I went to pay for the parking and looked at purchasing the monthly ticket Karen and Candy told me about.

This again saved me a small fortune instead of paying the daily parking fee. I had no idea how long we were going to be there waiting on a heart. I have heard some people have waited for months, some even years.

The evening was completed with my now "normal" takeaway dinner, a warm shower, a general update, and leaving messages for my friend, Brenda Hattingh in South Africa, who had started a small prayer group for Stan. She was such a blessing to me during this time.

Due to the time difference, we would leave voice notes when we could and catch up whenever we had time.

Friday, November 19, 2021

I spent the morning doing some research about accommodation as I needed to check out of the hotel by Sunday. To extend my stay in the same hotel, even on a longer-term basis worked out to around $150 per night and this was simply not an option. It would mean around $ 4,500 a month, just not possible for us.

Again, I had NO idea how long I would be in the city or how long to book for. It all depended on when a heart would become available and only God had the day and time for that appointment.

I looked at monthly apartment rentals which would be a lot cheaper, but most of them would only be available for the following month on. They would also be unfurnished and even though I would just need a bed, it was not a practical option.

I looked at other accommodation options online and found a place not too far from the hospital which was a sharing space, mostly with traveling nurses.

I am a private person and was not too keen on this but it was financially a much better option. Then came the burning question of how long I would need to book for.

I decided to book week by week at first and see how things go. At least I had a place to go for another week after Sunday when I needed to check out.

I also managed to make an appointment to have the noise on the car checked out at a service station close to the hotel. They could only fit me in early Monday morning but I was just too grateful they could help.

Candy, Karen, and I met early for coffee. They were like a breath of fresh air every time I saw them. Something familiar in a very unfamiliar situation.

We would bring each other up to date on the conditions of Dave and Stan and just have a few good laughs about silly things. We all needed laughs during this time and their humor was similar to mine.

We shared contact details and it was clear to me that I would have friends for a lifetime with these two ladies, not just during this time of facing challenges.

I was greeted with a "Good morning, honey," when I walked into Stan's room.

I sighed out loud in relief as at least I wasn't greeted by the same grumpy stranger from the day before. The miserable man.

He was less confused but there was still some confusion, none nearly as bad as the previous days.

"Have you spoken to Stew?" Stan asked.

"Yes, I speak to him every day to bring him up to date," I replied.

"Is he going to come to see me?" Stan asked.

Stewart lives in North Carolina and was tied up at work but he had called me to say he is going to make a plan. He wanted to surprise Stan.

"He is tied up at work but I am sure he will do his best," was my answer the almost twenty times Stan asked me that question over the next few hours.

"Maybe you and Stew could go watch the ballgame on Sunday if he is here because I don't think they will give me a pass," Stan said in all seriousness.

Yup, confusion still reigned but I couldn't help smiling as I now knew this would be temporary. He was also not nearly as agitated as the previous two days.

"I am going to be spending every minute I can with you handsome. I don't want to go watch ballgames. How about we watch it together on TV?" I suggested.

"Sounds good," he replied and pointed to what was left of his lunch, "Can you cut that for me, please?"

I was so grateful for a please and thank you from Stan again. The rude man that possessed him had left the building. Thank God!

Our afternoon was spent watching a little TV and Stan taking long naps while I spent my time staring out the window while sitting on my now favorite window seat.

The day turned out much better than the previous days and I felt I could breathe a little deeper again.

Saturday, November 20, 2021

I did some packing in the morning. This would be my last night in the hotel. I knew I would not get the same comfort from this point forward but I was so grateful for this blessing of the past week.

I followed my normal routine. Stopped at the store on the way to the hospital to get Stan his favorite yogurt and chocolate milk.

I had my coffee at the hospital while waiting for visiting hours. Each day was expecting the unexpected visiting Stan as his condition was different almost daily.

On this Saturday he seemed a little more at peace. It was a relief once again. His confusion was truly draining my energy and I found it hard to keep strong during his very confusing moments.

There was so much I was trying to deal with mentally and emotionally that his added confusion was a lot to bear.

I helped him with his lunch and decided to put the television on to distract him a little later in the afternoon. It was hard to hear with all the pumps and the HEPA filter but we managed.

Stan reached his hand towards me in a gesture to hold his hand. My husband was back! He allowed me to hold his hand again.

I flipped through the channels. "Tell me to stop when you see something you want to watch, ok?" I said.

I kept clicking through the channels slowly when Stan suddenly said, "I want to watch the cow."

My mind was racing. Cow? What cow? I didn't see a cow on any of the channels we just went through.

I started changing channels in reverse.

"Ok honey, I am going to go back. You tell me when you see the cow show," I said.

When I got to a children's animation movie he shouted with excitement, "There! That one. The cow! I want to watch the cow."

I burst out laughing. I was even a little surprised by the ugly laugh that I heard but I felt it from my gut and it was a small emotional release. Yes, that will be my excuse.

"Stan, that is called Ferdinand the Bull, he is not a cow," I laughed.

"Cow. Bull. What's the difference?" he smiled and continued watching.

The afternoon was spent holding hands and watching animation movies. Stan was back and the stranger had left the building. Thank God! He was no longer welcome here.

Sometime during the afternoon, a doctor from neurology visited Stan again and put an IV bag onto his line.

"What is that, doctor?" I asked.

"We are giving him a bit of sodium to help with the swelling and bleeding he had. This should help him," he explained.

Within minutes I could see and hear a change in Stan's behavior. He spoke more sense and the confusion was now leaving his body at a rapid rate. Thank you, Jesus! My husband was coming back to me.

After visiting hours, I went to the hotel to finish packing and called Stewart again to give him the good news about Stan doing better.

Sunday, November 21, 2021

I checked out of the hotel and decided to have a light lunch at the hospital as I could only book into the new place after 3 p.m.

I spent the afternoon making Stan as comfortable as possible, helping him with his meals, and watching a few shows with him.

When he fell asleep I would have my seat in the window and watch the world happen outside. It seemed like everything was in slow motion and strangely it relaxed me.

I left the hospital a little earlier to go check in at the new place. It had A LOT of stairs and I had quite a bit of luggage. I didn't want to leave anything in the car as this was not a secure hotel parking lot.

I finally made it, everything was safe in my room. I settled in quickly before heading downstairs to put a few things in the fridge.

I had my private bedroom but there was a shared bathroom, kitchen, and lounge. This was shared with two other bedroom occupants.

While I was making something to eat I heard a voice behind me, "Hi, are you the new lady?"

I turned around and saw a strong-looking guy smiling at me.

"Hi, yes I just came in a few minutes ago," I said. "I'm Liesl Gregory," and I stretched my hand out to him for a handshake.

"Nice to meet you, I am Ogaga Uhrie," he said as he shook my hand.

"Ogaga Uhrie? Gosh with a name like that and that accent you sound like someone from Africa somewhere?" I said.

He laughed and said, "Yes I am, I am from Nigeria but I moved to the US quite a few years ago when my parents moved to West Virginia. You don't sound American either?" he said.

"No, I am from South Africa but I have been here since 2018," I explained.

We immediately connected and it was like God sent me a "familiar face" from the same continent in this time of unknown and unfamiliarity.

Ogaga explained he is a resident doctor at the hospital and rented there full-time. The other room was currently empty and he was happy to have someone around.

We spent the evening getting to know each other while eating dinner. I noticed a few puzzle boxes stacked on the end of the long dining room table.

We discovered we both found building puzzles very relaxing and continued to start a new puzzle while sharing about ourselves.

I told him about Stan and he promised to come and visit us in the MICU the next day. He was doing a surgical residency.

I went to bed thanking God for the new friend. This African friend found me across countries during a time I needed someone familiar more than ever before.

Ogaga was light during a dark, unknown time. He was my lighthouse. A man with a heart of gold and with an incredible passion for helping people.

Monday, November 22, 2021

I was up early to get the car to the service station. They were going to do their best to have my car fixed by 1 p.m. so I could visit Stan at 2 p.m. I explained the situation and Mohammed, the owner, was super accommodating.

He gave me a comfortable space to sit while I waited and kept me updated on what they found with the car. I had a few hours to catch up on updates with all communications and also to browse for new accommodations for the following week.

At noon Mohammed came to me and said they fixed the problem but when they removed the tires he noticed my back brakes needed to be replaced. They were in very bad shape from the salt roads back home from the winter roads on snow days.

He didn't seem like the kind of guy to try to rip people off but I was cautious that it was not just a dealer trying to make an extra unnecessary buck off a vulnerable woman.

He seemed sincere when he said he didn't want me to drive with the brakes the way it was. I also needed the car to be safe.

I explained that I needed to be at the hospital by 2 p.m. and asked if I would make it. I suddenly felt overwhelmed. Mohammed assured me they will work fast and do their best.

Roughly another half an hour later he came to me and said, "The car is not going to be ready in time so I am going to arrange a taxi for you. A guy I know and use often, not a stranger, to take you to the hospital."

"I will arrange for him to fetch you again at 6 pm from the hospital. I will leave the car keys with my son at the service station right next door. I will pay for the taxi. I do not want you to miss the visit with your husband," he said.

I was blown away by his kindness and generosity. He knew I was from out of town and that Stan was very ill, waiting on a transplant.

Being the emotional wreck I was, I started crying, feeling so overwhelmed by this stranger's kindness.

He kept saying, "Don't cry, you will see your husband and I will fix the car, ok? I will call you when it is done but the driver will fetch you again at 6 p.m. and bring you here."

I was so utterly grateful but this was NYC and there was a part of me that was nervous about having to trust a stranger. This was a lot of trust, but I handed it to God and He knew, so He sent yet another stranger to reassure me.

A lady came and sat next to me as I waited for the driver and she started to speak to me. She said she brought her car in for an inspection and she doesn't trust anyone other than Mohammed and his team.

"So he is trustworthy?" I asked her again.

"Oh, absolutely!" she said and at that moment I felt total peace.

God sent me reassurance, He knows my heart.

The taxi driver fetched me at 1 pm and took me to the hospital. I started speaking to the driver and he said he does a lot of driving for Mohammed.

"I have been driving customers for Mohammed for years now, since I first came to the USA from Africa," he said.

Are you kidding me? What are the chances? God was just reassuring me I was in His hands every step of the journey by sending me another friend from Africa.

It was so good to spend time with Stan again that afternoon and he was a lot less confused. The heart team explained that once Stan gets out of the fourteen day quarantine from COVID, he would be moved to the area where other patients are awaiting transplants. He had another six days to go!

At 6 p.m. my driver picked me up again and took me back to the service station. Mohammed's son gave me my keys and the invoice. Mohammed never charged me for installing the breaks, only for the parts. Yet another blessing during this time.

I cried all the way while driving to my temporary home. I felt so spoiled by God. I was experiencing God's favor daily.

The car drove like a dream, with no noise whatsoever. I turned the volume up of the song playing on the radio, crying while singing along.

Goodness of God

Bethel Music

I love You, Lord
Oh Your mercy never fails me
All my days
I've been held in Your hands
From the moment that I wake up
Until I lay my head
Oh I will sing of the goodness of God

All my life You have been faithful
All my life You have been so so good
With every breath that I am able
Oh I will sing of the goodness of God

I love Your voice
You have led me through the fire
In the darkest night
You are close like no other
I've known You as a Father
I've known You as a friend
I have lived in the goodness of God
Oh

And all my life You have been faithful
All my life You have been so so good
With every breath that I am able

Oh I will sing of the goodness of God

Yeah yeah yeah
'Cause Your goodness is running, it's running after me
Your goodness is running, it's running after me
With my life laid down, I'm surrendered now, I give You everything
Your goodness is running, it's running after me

Your goodness is running, it's running after me
Your goodness is running, it's running after me
With my life laid down, I'm surrendered now, I give You everything
Your goodness is running, it keeps running after me

All my life You have been faithful
All my life You have been so so good
With every breath that I am able
Oh I will sing of the goodness of God
I'm gonna sing, I'm gonna sing

And all my life You have been faithful
All my life You have been so so good
With every breath that I am able
Oh I will sing of the goodness of God
I'm gonna sing of the goodness of God

I was singing about surrendering but I had no idea how total surrender to God in a few days would change things dramatically.

At "home" I joined Ogaga and we had a meal together sharing about our days while we built a puzzle to relax.

He apologized for not coming to see me and Stan in the MICU that day but he was overwhelmed with cases and promised to pop in the following day.

Tuesday, November 23, 2021

Stewart called to say he was going to surprise Stan on the 25th for Thanksgiving Day. He found a place to stay close to the hotel for a night or two.

I knew it would be tough on me to keep it a surprise. Stan was asking me daily if Stew was planning on coming to see him.

I took some time in the morning and went shopping for Stan for some basics as I forgot his bag in the lounge next to the couch when I left home in such a rush just over a week ago.

He didn't need much and I thought I would start with a few toiletries and underwear. Other things I could get on the next trip to the store.

After my mini shopping spree, I ran into Candy and Karen before visiting hours and it was great to catch up. Dave was getting better slowly, but there was steady improvement.

They were excited to hear about Stan's improvement and Karen couldn't wait to share the news with Dave.

There wasn't much change in Stan when I got to his room. A little confusion but a lot less than it was a few days earlier.

Dr. Lanier came in and asked Stan a couple of general questions.

"Do you know what hospital you are at Mr. Gregory?" he asked Stan. "No," he replied.

Dr. Lanier looked at me concerned and said, "he didn't know the name yesterday either."

I giggled and said, "Doc, that's Stan. If a name is too hard for him to pronounce he simply doesn't."

"Westchester is like saying Worcestershire sauce to him. Too hard so he doesn't even try. You should ask him anything else," I said and the serious Doctor Lanier even cracked a smile which I could see even through the double mask and face shield.

"Ok then I will be asking you some new questions," he said laughing. "Mr. Gregory, I am happy with things right now. The brain bleed is under control and neurology has signed you off as good for a transplant, I am sure they have told you this," he continued.

"Great," Stan responded.

It was a relief knowing Stan was listed but, again, we knew there was a long unknown road ahead. No one knew when a heart would become available to Stan and I remember too clearly how Dr. Lanier explained Stan might need hospice if he doesn't get listed, and receive a heart in time.

During the rest of the afternoon, I watched poor Nurse Andrew having to deal with the balloon pump alarm almost every 30 minutes.

He had to reset it each time and said it is working but the alarm keeps going off. He called the heart team to come look at it.

Ogaga came to visit Stan and it was so wonderful to introduce the two. I had told Stan about Ogaga and it was good for them both to be able to put a face to the name. He stayed for a little while till he was called again for another emergency surgery.

Nurse Andrew later came back into the room with another doctor who had a look at the balloon pump machine next to Stan's bed.

They spoke amongst themselves and the doctor turned to us and said, "It seems there is an issue with this balloon."

"We will have to take Mr. Gregory to have a new one set. I am going to see when the soonest we can take him and will let you know, ok Mr. Gregory?" he explained.

"I'll be here," Stan said calmly.

Just before the end of visiting hours, they fetched Stan to replace the balloon pump.

I felt so sorry for Stan as he already had so many procedures but he took it like a true champ.

Surgeries and procedures were nothing new to Stan. On September 26, 2020, on our wedding day, Stan was rushed to the Emergency room with compartment syndrome in his arm due to the blood thinners from the failing heart.

He had slightly torn a muscle in his bicep a few days earlier and due to the blood thinners, he kept bleeding into the arm cavity till his arm was double the size and bruised from his shoulder down to his wrist.

He was misdiagnosed twice before he was taken to Rochester General Hospital after he collapsed in the car park after the wedding ceremony.

They did emergency surgery on him to save his arm, and his life, according to the surgeon. He was in the hospital on a wound vacuum pump as they could not close the arm after surgery due to the swelling.

He was in the hospital for three weeks till they could finally close the wound with a skin graft from his leg. Personally I believe this was a big blow to his failing heart at the time.

So Stan had walked a few miles when it came to procedures but this latest journey was a completely new kettle of fish.

I decided to go back to the guest house as the procedure would take longer than what visiting hours would allow.

Stan called me later to say all went well and he is back in the room and the new pump has not alarmed so all seemed good.

I was excited as the hospital changed its visiting hours from the following day. I would be able to see Stan from 11 a.m. to 9 p.m.

As I went to sleep that night I was reminded that it was only two weeks earlier that I dropped Stan off at Rochester General Hospital ED. So much had happened over 14 days, it felt like 14 months.

During the evening and throughout the night, I had about five more calls from Stan.

I think it was a combination of ICU delirium, boredom, needing to be reassured he is not alone, and being woken up every time someone came to do bloodwork or check IVs.

I struggled to get decent rest being woken up so often and taking time to fall asleep again, but I knew I was Stan's lifeline and not answering was not even an option. Not at all.

Wednesday, November 24, 2021

First thing in the morning, I asked the owner of the guesthouse I was currently staying in if I could extend my stay.

Unfortunately, the room was already booked by a traveling nurse for a few weeks. I would have to search and find the next place to stay, but I needed to get to the hospital early for the earlier visiting hours.

Stan was doing well but he was struggling with anxiety, especially at night. Understandably so. The neurologist was confident that the brain bleed had resolved and that the last bit of confusion would be a part of history soon.

I was excited about Stewart coming to see Stan the next day, I was desperate for a familiar family face myself and I knew Stan would be over the moon as he had been asking for Stew for days.

It was almost impossible to keep the secret to surprise Stan. But I did, I wanted to see the surprise on Stan's face when Stew walked in.

Medically, our next goal at this stage was to get Stan out of isolation from the positive COVID test. We only had a few days to go but it felt like weeks.

During times like this, your best bet to cope is to break things into the smallest little goals. This way you feel that you are moving forward even if it's with small steps.

After the day's visit, I went "home" to go find yet another "home" for the next few weeks. At least now I knew Stan was listed and that meant a huge step forward. I focused on the positive.

I found a place through a website that was available from Sunday afternoon when I needed to be out of my current space.

I booked it until the 8th of January. I knew Stan would be in hospital till at least then and this way I didn't have to find a place or move around over Christmas and New Year.

The constant moving was tiring me out and I was looking forward to calling a space "home" for a little while longer than a week.

I was a little nervous about the place, though, as it looked so beautiful on the website and it was so reasonably priced compared to other places. Once again, I had to put it into God's hands.

I had Stew's visit to look forward to the next day for Thanksgiving. This was definitely a different way of celebrating Thanksgiving. There would be no turkey dinner with family but our situation gave me a new perspective of giving thanks.

CHAPTER 5

Thanksgiving

Thursday, November 25, 2021

Thanksgiving Day. I felt there was so much to be thankful for even though we were living a life of blind faith in so many ways.

The hospital had an outside person who brought all the patients listed for heart transplants a special Thanksgiving meal and they didn't forget about Stan in the MICU.

It was such a blessing to give Stan some turkey, gravy, vegetables, corn and so many other things overflowing on this plate of bliss.

Shortly after he finished some lunch, Stewart messaged me that he was downstairs in the hospital lobby. I told Stan I needed a quick coffee break and went to fetch Stewart.

We both geared up and Stan didn't notice us in the hallway. At this time Stan was still oblivious to the fact that Stewart was going to surprise him and was asking me almost every day if I knew if Stewart was going to come to see him.

When we walked into the room Stan looked up, saw me, and looked to see who was following behind me. It was hard to recognize anyone with a double mask, face shield, and hairnet.

Stan had the look on his face of total confusion that turned to disbelief when Stewart spoke.

"Now what did you do, Stanley?" Stew asked loud as he stepped closer to the bed.

Stan's face just lit up! He knew that voice.

What a beautiful Thanksgiving gift. The two bantered like they always do. Stewart pretended to pull some of the machine's power cords and Stan pretended to press the emergency bell to call the nurse to rescue him from Stew.

I gave the two some alone brother time and they promised not to try and escape or burn the place down while I went to have a break downstairs in the coffee shop.

About an hour or so later I headed back up to the MICU. As I walked through the double doors I saw all the families visiting but sadly people were limited to two visitors due to COVID.

Even though it was a holiday there were no fewer staff or patients in the MICU. I looked into the rooms as I passed wondering what each patient was struggling with.

As I stood outside Stan's room I watched him and Stew bantering and it was so good to see Stan laughing with just so much joy that filled the room.

The two brothers are very close and there is never a dull moment with the two together.

Later in the evening, Stewart and I had a small dinner in the hospital coffee shop. We could catch up on everything Stan was going through.

It was such a blessing to have him there for support for a couple of days and simply download everything.

Friday, November 26, 2021

I once again had multiple calls from Stan throughout the night. It was clear he was suffering from ICU delirium. He didn't realize that if he was awake at 2 a.m. it didn't mean I was.

I would take every call. Almost every hour. There was no way I would not answer. I was his lifeline.

When I arrived at the hospital there were a few people in his room busy doing tests to see if Stan had a blood clot in his leg. His one foot became quite cold and they were concerned about blood flow to the leg and foot.

They didn't find any blood clots, thank the Lord. Looking back it was due to his heart deteriorating so rapidly that the blood supply became weaker and weaker in his extremities making it feel cold.

Stewart visited with Stan again and it was again the highlight of Stan's day. Late afternoon Stew had to leave to get back to North Carolina and still had a 10 hour drive ahead of him.

It was a sad goodbye and I think both Stew and Stan realized this might be the last time they see each other but they were both too proud to say the words and both holding onto faith that Stan was going to be ok.

They both felt they needed to be strong for the other. Funny how in a space like that, you do not want to look like you have lost hope, but you also do not want to pretend things do not look too rosy at the time.

Saturday, November 27, 2021

I met Candy and Karen for coffee before visiting hours and just enjoyed their company so much. The laughs, the familiar faces.

We got along so well and they started feeling like family to me. They were excited that Stan could soon be moved from Medical ICU to Cardiac ICU.

It was day 14 of Stan's COVID isolation and we were praying for a negative test result so he could finally move to the Cardiac ICU and feel less like a leper.

It would mean less gear for visitors and he would be able to see the faces easier.

Karen's boyfriend, Dave, was still in ICU but was slowly doing better. It was clear during this time that people in ICU need family support. Someone to advocate for them in a way as they are too weak to be able to do so for themselves.

At 11 a.m. we took the elevator to the second floor. We walked up to the Medical ICU entrance and rang the bell on the intercom.

A gentleman was waiting at the door as we arrived. He mentioned he rang the bell a few minutes ago and was still waiting for someone to respond.

The four of us stood there sharing a moment. All four of us waited for the double doors to open so we could get to our loved ones.

The man looked stressed but I didn't find it strange. Most visitors at ICU are under stress as their loved ones are in critical condition.

The doors finally opened and the gentleman walked ahead. He took a right into one of the first rooms to the right and I caught a glimpse of a lady laying on her back with breathing tubes.

She wasn't moving and I could see life support machines. Things didn't look well for her. That moment, that image was etched into my mind.

It was her birthday. There were no celebrations that day.

It is strange how we experience moments of interaction with strangers and never even realize how significant the moment could be. God had a plan. He is a God of details. Just how much detail, I would uncover months later.

When I got to Stan's room there was excitement in the room. The nurse said she kept pressing the refresh button on the test results on the system.

She was waiting on the results of the COVID test she did on Stan early that morning.

Finally, around 11 a.m. the result came in. NEGATIVE! Hallelujah! We all celebrated by ripping off our face shields, gloves, gowns, and hairnets. We were celebrating while a family was grieving for someone on her birthday down the hallway.

It was the longest fourteen days ever with Stan in COVID quarantine. I was so grateful that during this time, almost two weeks after visiting Stan, I kept testing negative and was able to continue seeing him.

I became a well-known face at the test station by now and I would joke as I pulled up saying, "good morning ladies and gentleman, I am here for another negative COVID test."

The one male, the only male, that worked at the testing drive-through, John, was such a pleasure and eventually greeted me by saying, "Morning, Mrs. Gregory. I have your negative test ready, we just need to swab your brain through your nose."

It was those little things that became little highlights in a world that had become so small yet overwhelming. Living life almost hour by hour.

As long as I kept taking stacks of Vitamin C, Zinc, Vitamin D and other vitamins I seemed to keep strong enough to keep the COVID virus at bay. Who am I kidding? All the glory to God! He was my protector.

Within a couple of hours of celebrating Stan's freedom from COVID, a room became available for him in the Cardiac ICU. It was time to pack his things and move to the 4th-floor. Going up!

Stan's new room was super small and had no window, but he was not a leper anymore and people didn't need to wear anything other than a mask into his room. Most importantly he was now in the wing he was meant to be in.

The medical plan at this time was to have him in this Cardiac ICU until they could move the balloon pump from the groin to the armpit, also known as auxiliary.

This way he would be able to get up and move, even walk around while pushing the pump machine along. He would feel more free in the transplant patient waiting unit being to walk around.

They planned to do the surgery on Monday as it was not an emergency and only emergency surgeries would be done on the weekend.

It wasn't like we were in a particular rush to get anywhere either so a couple of days would be no issue.

We continued to celebrate his freedom from isolation with a takeout meal from the coffee shop. Stan's favorite. Mac and Cheese with added broccoli to make him feel less guilty.

We had a reasonably peaceful day and I left the hospital to go pack my things once again for the move the following day. It was good to spend the last few hours at the guest house with my friend Ogaga.

He blessed me with a few puzzles to keep me occupied in the new guesthouse. We made sure we shared all contact details and knew we would keep contact in the future. We had a connection, a special friendship.

Before I went to sleep I did the general updates on Stan's condition and it was truly amazing to get prayer from my friend Brenda back in South Africa. She was such a prayer warrior for me and Stan during this time.

Stan's good friend, Mike Yodice, also kept checking in on Stan and me and it was so appreciated. It became clear he was also walking a close road with Jesus.

God was showing me how He is a God of details in this time. His goodness was not running but chasing after me.

CHAPTER 6

Total Surrender

Sunday, November 28, 2021

This day turned out to be very significant in Stan's future but I only learned about that much later in 2022.

It was a moving day for me once again. I carried all my goods down all the stairs once more and loaded the car with everything I owned down in the Big Apple.

Candy and Karen met me, yet again, for coffee and our morning updates on our loved ones. It was good to hear there was a constant improvement with Dave.

When I arrived at Stan's room, it was a pleasant surprise to see him alert and awake.

Even though Stan was now in a room with no window and constant lights, a recipe for ICU delirium, he was more alert than I had seen him in a while.

We had some morning entertainment from the guy across the hallway who was screaming and shouting at the hospital staff and eventually threatened them. He looked like a gang member and certainly acted like one.

He was soon moved to another unit as they didn't want to expose all the patients to the drama. This meant we had to watch television for the remainder of the day. No more live entertainment.

The nurses were in and out all day doing blood work, checking on the IVs and balloon pump. Stan had his usual naps and I would venture out for a coffee.

Candy and Karen messaged me and asked if I wanted to meet for lunch in the coffee shop. Stan said I should go as he would just doze off for a while and I needed a break.

It was so wonderful to hear about Dave's improvements. He was obviously a fighter and thank God for Karen and Candy who were fighting for him all the way.

These two ladies were such a blessing in my life at the time. I do not think they realize just how much to this day.

Later in the day, after spending a few hours with Stan, I said my goodbyes for the night a little earlier than normal.

I needed to go and find my new home, 15 minutes' drive from the hospital and I didn't want to get lost in the dark.

I drove to the new place hoping and praying it would be what I saw in the photos or at least close to it. I was told I would be the only person in the house as the owner only recently bought the place and has only set up the main bedroom and en-suite for guests.

They were not living in the house themselves so I would have the entire place to myself.

Thank God for GPS and I found the place in good time. The house was beautiful from the outside. I had instructions from the owner about how to gain access and where everything was located.

I walked through the front door. It was as beautiful as the pictures showed, even prettier. What a relief! I took a right, up the few stairs, and walked to the room at the end of the hallway, the master bedroom.

When I opened the door I could not believe what I saw. I dropped my bag I had over my shoulder and fell to my knees.

I burst into tears. It was the most beautiful room I had ever seen. The décor was spectacularly beautiful. An on-suite to die for. A huge dressing room.

I was on my knees in gratitude to God for giving me this space for the next few weeks. When I finally stopped crying enough so I could see properly I noticed a wooden basket of goodies on the chair with a note.

"You take care of your husband, I will take care of you," it read.

In the basket were so many treats. From a super soft gown, socks, a notebook, bubble baths, energy bars, and so much more things.

I was dumbstruck. "Lord, you are so good to me. You are such a good Father! THANK YOU," I prayed as I sat down on the edge of the big bed with crisp white linen, and I continued crying.

I felt so incredibly spoiled at that moment. I went to see the rest of the house and brought in all my luggage from the car. I messaged the owner to say thank you and that her kindness had me in tears.

From her correspondence, I could gather she was a believer as well. Blessing upon blessing. I later learned she is an ordained minister and she asked if she could put Stan on their group prayer chat. Is God good or what?

Besides having a beautiful home to stay in, I finally had a kitchen where I could make decent meals and a fridge I could put some groceries in.

There was a laundry area to do washing. The lounge was beautifully furnished with a huge television mounted to the wall next to the fireplace.

It was such a tranquil space. A space I could now come "home" to and relax when I came back from the hospital at night.

I was overflowing with gratitude during the toughest time of my life. God is good. All the time!

Monday, November 29, 2021

I was eager to get to the hospital to share the incredible news with Stan and show him the photos I took of all the rooms.

First I had to go shopping for some groceries and also to stock up on some of Stan's favorite things.

Protein shakes, high protein yogurt, chocolate, and chocolate milk. There was now a big fridge I could keep things in and didn't have to worry about being considerate to other people. The space was mine.

By visiting time I walked into the hospital lobby and I was greeted by Candy and Karen and their beautiful smiles. These two ladies always smiled. I shared my news and they celebrated with me.

Stan looked good when I walked into his room. He got a big smile when he saw the treats and quickly finished off a protein drink. He didn't particularly like hospital food. Who does?

He told me the doctor said they would do the balloon move on Tuesday so we could relax for the day. Waiting was going to be our friend for a while anyways.

I broke away for a quick cup of coffee with Candy and Karen sometime during the day.

"I told Dave about Stan and he is happy to hear he is doing better," Karen said with a big smile.

"Stan also asked about you guys today so we will have to let the guys meet sometime in the future," I said.

"Absolutely," Candy said.

It was clear a friendship was developing and these ladies started creeping deep into my heart.

I got Stan a treat meal again for dinner before I left from the coffee shop. Mac and cheese, he would eat it each day given the opportunity, with a protein shake.

He was nil-per-mouth from midnight that night for the surgery the next day so he made up for not having breakfast the following morning and had a really good dinner.

On the way home I kept thanking God for the space I was going to. I made dinner, a healthy dinner, not a quick box dinner, and spent some time watching a television show.

I got into the hot tub and sat there crying while singing worship songs just praising God for his goodness. There is something magical about living in the favor of God.

Tuesday, November 30, 2021

We were not sure what time Stan would go in for surgery but he would call when he was given a time. By the time I got to the hospital for visiting hours, he was still waiting to receive news.

By lunchtime, I asked the nurse to check on the timing again as Stan was dying for a drink of water. He had not had anything since midnight.

She came back after a few minutes and said, "He can have something to drink and I am ordering him some food now."

"The doctor just told us that they cannot fit him in today as it is not an emergency," she explained.

"Fair enough, but could you confirm when it would be done then?" I asked.

"The doctor will come and speak to you in a minute, he is around," she said.

In later months I would learn there was a reason for these details. As I said, God is a God of details. There is no such thing as a coincidence when you are a believer. God is always in control and every detail of this miracle was unfolding.

Not long after, a doctor came into the room and explained that since Stan's surgery is not an emergency they could not fit him in for the day but he was confirmed for 8 a.m. the following morning.

I didn't have an issue about it as there was no rush and we chose to look at it from a point of view that these surgeons might be doing transplants for patients who might have been blessed with a donor heart.

Stan made up for the breakfast he missed and had a double lunch, followed by a good rest when he had satisfied his hunger and thirst. We watched some television and I shared some photos of the place I was staying at.

Stan was relieved to see I was taken care of and that I would be there for a while not needing to move again till at least January 8th.

I explained that I could extend the stay later when we had a better indication of the timeline.

The waiting game on a donor organ is a mental battle when you are on a transplant list. You NEVER know when you will get that call. It could be today, tomorrow, or nine months from today.

All I knew was my husband would not make it for months, or even one month for that matter. It was in God's hands. Even though he had moments of looking really good it was the balloon pump and medications which helped and these were temporary solutions.

Often people on the transplant list and their families struggle during this time. Then there is false guilt which many also need to face.

I call it false because it is a type of guilt you should not be carrying, yet many do. A feeling of, "I am waiting for someone to die so I can live."

For patients waiting on an organ, the donor's death has nothing to do with the need for a new organ. That person has an appointment with God. We all do and God is the only one that knows that date and time.

The donor is going to leave this earth and leave a body behind. A body which might have organs someone in need could use for a few more years.

The need for an organ doesn't cause someone to die. These donors are heroes for leaving their bodies to be used, allowing someone else to live.

I believed the heart that God wanted Stan to have would be available in God's time. Divine timing. At that time, He will be meeting with the donor. An appointment no one has control over.

This is not organ trafficking where people die so others can live. This is a legal system, a process with so much respect for the donor and the recipient.

Every time I thought about this I would pray for the donor and their family, often crying while doing so. I felt like I could feel the sorrow they were going to face.

The enemy hated the fact that Stan was doing well, all considering, and that God was working a miracle. We know the enemy comes to steal, kill and destroy.

"It" tried to stop this miracle in any possible way but God won this battle long ago. We needed to stay faithful and never give up.

On one of my breaks I ran into Dr. Lanier in the hallway of the ICU. "I am happy to see Stan in the Cardiac ICU and on the transplant list. I need to contact his insurance as they declined a possible transplant," he said.

"What? NO! Why? After all this? Now that he is listed?" I said.

"Don't worry. I know why and I will sort it out," he explained.

"Why doctor?" I asked.

"They saw on the record he had a brain bleed so, therefore, they denied a transplant thinking he might not recover from the bleed, but I need to just let them know he has recovered and neurology has signed him off," he explained.

The stress was unbearable. This was a roller coaster for sure. Just when you think you have hit the bottom of the big dipper suddenly you start climbing again and you haven't even got your breath back.

Dr. Lanier worked his magic and got the insurance to approve a possible transplant again.

That evening I followed my new ritual. Get "home." Make dinner. Have a bath or shower, and watch a bit of television before bed, after all the updates.

That evening's update read:

"Today was a little frustrating but adding to our teaching of patience and the big horrible word called… *Waiting*! Stan's auxiliary balloon has been postponed to tomorrow morning at 8 a.m."

I sat in the living room while waiting for dinner to finish in the oven and had the television on. I just couldn't find anything watchable so I switched to YouTube and searched "worship videos."

I pressed play on the first one that came up.

The next moment I had an experience I never had before and I could never have imagined.

The song, "I Surrender" by Hillsong started playing. I immediately felt incredibly emotional. I found myself on my knees, arms stretched into the air singing along on top of my lungs.

"I surrender to the Lord. I surrender Stan, the situation, and our worries to you Lord," I prayed.

Then, suddenly I had a beautiful vision.

Jesus was sitting next to Stan on a park bench behind the hospital building. I was standing at a distance so I could not hear the conversation but could see them and "knew" what the conversation was about. Jesus was speaking to Stan.

Stan became emotional. He started crying and Jesus put His arm on Stan's back. Stan started weeping. Jesus spoke to Stan about his "old life." The life he was about to leave behind.

Stan dropped his head into his hands and his elbows into his knees, he cried uncontrollably. Jesus stood up, knelt in front of Stan, and then started to wash his feet. Stan continued crying. When Jesus was done washing Stan's feet, he got up and sat down next to Stan again. Jesus put his arm around Stan once more. Consoling him.

Jesus said something to him and they both laughed. Stan stopped crying and laughed through the tears.

Jesus washed the old Stan's life away and it was now a new Stan. They both stood up and Jesus hugged Stan. They walked back into the hospital, Jesus with his hand still on Stan's back, showing total support.

"I SURRENDER LORD," I kept saying. There was a peace I cannot describe that came over me. A peace that I had never felt before. I was weeping and managed to finally control my emotion enough to take a decent deep breath.

I Surrender

Hillsong Worship

Here I am
Down on my knees again
Surrendering all
Surrendering all

And find me here
Lord as You draw me near
I'm desperate for You
I'm desperate for You
I surrender

Drench my soul
As mercy and grace unfold
I hunger and thirst
I hunger and thirst

With arms stretched wide
I know You hear my cry
Speak to me now
Speak to me now

I surrender
I surrender
I want to know You more
I want to know You more

I surrender
I surrender
I want to know You more
I want to know You more

Like a rushing wind
Jesus breathe within
Lord have Your way
Lord have Your way in me
Like a mighty storm
Stir within my soul
Lord have Your way
Lord have Your way in me

Like a rushing wind
Jesus breathe within
Lord have Your way
Lord have Your way in me
Like a mighty storm
Stir within my soul
Lord have Your way
Lord have Your way in me

Like a rushing wind
Jesus breathe within
Lord have Your way
Lord have Your way in me (like a mighty storm)
Like a mighty storm
Stir within my soul

Lord have Your way
Lord have Your way in me
Lord have Your way
Lord have Your way in me

I surrender
I surrender
I want to know You more
I want to know You more
I surrender
I surrender
I want to know You more
I want to know You more.
I wasn't sure what I just witnessed all meant but I knew God was in control.

I surrendered. TOTALLY. It was no longer, "Jesus take the wheel so I could get into the back seat, but Jesus take the wheel, take the car, take everything and please take it where it is meant to go."

I handed my life and Stan's life to God that night. I put all our worries and concerns onto a serving tray and handed the tray to God. I lay there on the floor in total vulnerability to God. Total faith. Releasing all control I had wanted to hang onto.

I went to sleep with peace in my heart. I wanted to get to the hospital as early as I could so I would be there when Stan's surgery was done and share what I had experienced, what I saw.

Never in my wildest dreams could I have imagined what was about to happen.

CHAPTER 7

Miracles

Wednesday, December 1, 2021

At 7.55 a.m. my phone rang. It was Stan. Why is he calling? He should be in the OR. Is something wrong? Did they postpone the surgery, again?

"Hey. What's up?" I answered.

"Morning, is this Mrs. Gregory?" a voice said.

"Yes, who is this?" I was concerned.

"This is Dr. Levine. I just wanted to let you know I have some good news. We have a heart for Stan," he said.

"WHAT???" I yelled.

Through a gasp of relief, I heard Dr. Levine say again, "We have a heart for Stan. We are looking at doing the surgery at noon.

We had an offer very early this morning and Stan looks like a great match and it is a healthy heart," he explained.

I could hardly speak. Thirteen days listed and there is a donor heart for Stan. A HEALTHY heart clear of hepatitis.

"Stan hasn't had anything to eat as he would have gone for the balloon so he is in perfect shape for the surgery in a few hours," Dr. Levine continued.

I was dumbstruck. God-smacked.

"Why don't you come through to the hospital now and spend some time with him before he goes in? I will arrange for you to come in early," Dr. Levine said.

I must have said, "Thank you thank you thank you," twenty times as I had no other words.

When I hung up I became emotional. An emotion of gratitude and overwhelming sadness knowing there is a donor family heartbroken about a loved one who has passed away.

There are no words for these emotions. This is not something experienced enough for some intellectual person to have manufactured a vocabulary for these emotions.

I prayed for the donor. For the donor's family and the grief they were facing. I then changed my focus back to my husband. He needed me now more than ever and I needed to get to the hospital as quickly as possible.

I called Stew, Zaan and Taylor, and Mike on the way to the hospital. When I arrived at the front desk in the lobby I explained my husband was going in for a transplant and Dr. Levine arranged early access for me.

They didn't know about this and tried to call the ICU to find out more details. The next moment the elevator opens and Dr. Levine walks out. Details! God's details!

This man always appeared at the right time and was proving again what a blessing he was in our lives. Earth Angel for sure!

Dr. Levine spotted me and started walking toward me.
"Doc, they won't let me in," I said.

He looked at the person behind the counter and with authority in his voice he said, "This lady's husband is having a heart transplant and she needs to get through and to his room right now please."

He turned to me and continued to explain that they are aiming for surgery at noon but will keep me updated. I could sense the excitement in his voice.

I could not get to Stan's room quick enough. It was a small room but today there was almost no space for me to step inside. There were so many people around his bed, I felt claustrophobic on his behalf.

Most of the transplant team was there. The anesthetist, surgeons, nurses, man it felt like even the janitors had a meeting there in that room right then.

I wiggled myself a spot at the bottom end of Stan's bed and he noticed me immediately.

"Hey honey," he said and everyone looked over at me.

"Hey you, you're getting a heart!!" I said excitedly and tried not to become too emotional but was exploding inside.

I struggled to contain myself.

Everyone in the room who didn't know me now knew who I was and bombarded me with questions. Stan was overwhelmed and they wanted to confirm some things with me.

A doctor standing next to me looked at me and asked, "Is your husband vaccinated?"

I wanted to slap him at that moment. Seriously doctor. Firstly, who are you? I have never seen you before.

Secondly, Can you not read his chart? If you are a doctor then you should have access to his charts?

Thirdly, why ask me *now*? Now that we are about to go to the OR for a heart transplant? Was there no opportunity to ask me this earlier, maybe in the weeks we have been here?

I got instantly annoyed but thankfully none of my thoughts escaped my mouth. I was not going to allow this man to steal our moment, our joy.

As politely as I could I said, "No."

He mumbled and said, "It's too late now," and then continued to ask me, "Have you been vaccinated?"

The dear Lord restrained me. I wanted to scream! SERIOUSLY!? Now?

"NO! I am not. Neither is he," I said as calmly as I could, but I know it came out annoyed, and I quickly moved my focus to Stan.

I heard him say as I was turning to Stan, "Well, you will have to get vaccinated TODAY!"

He felt like a little porch-pooping dog trying to bite at my heels while I tried to focus on something much more important.

For the sake of not creating a scene I simply replied. "Sure!" and moved my focus to the doctor's present who would be in the OR with my husband in a few hours.

Trying to focus on the moment and what was actually about to happen. My husband was about to have a heart transplant!

I think he might have "felt" my irritation with him and he left the room, probably for his own safety as I was not going to have any more from this stranger.

This doctor, who could not even introduce himself to me, wanting to simply vaccinate people, left a sour taste in my mouth.

He didn't even know my name, my medical condition, nothing. He simply wanted to wipe his vaccine on someone he knows nothing about.

As the important questions were answered from all the other staff members in the room, they all slowly filtered out the room as they were satisfied with the answers to their questions.

Finally! I got to speak to Stan. I kissed him and we were both at a lack of words for the incredibly quick wait we had.

I had to shave Stan's three-week-old beard as they preferred him clean-shaven for surgery. I was so nervous. I knew if I broke his skin in any way he might not get the heart.

It might sound ridiculous but I was a quick study in all the details of precautions taken by the heart transplant team.

When a patient receives an organ their immune system is shut down, suppressed, and they are prone to infection so if they have sores or broken skin this could count against them in being considered.

My poor husband got a very patchy shave but no nicks.

Doctors and nurses kept flooding in and out of the room. At 11 a.m. we were informed that surgery was to be expected at 3 p.m.

My immediate thoughts went to the donor's family once again. This must be the time they say their goodbyes and my thoughts and prayers immediately went out to them.

I could not imagine the heartbreak they are experiencing during this time. I had to keep my focus on Stan and be positive even though it was hard as an empath not to sense their pain.

We finally got a moment where it was just the two of us in the room.

I leaned over and asked him, "How do you feel?"

I saw a look in his eyes I had never seen before. "Scared," he replied.

"I would be worried if you weren't scared, it is completely understandable," I said.

I took my phone and searched for the worship song "I Surrender" and started playing it for Stan.

"Stan, God has got you. He promised me he was going to perform a miracle in your life. It's happening.

My God, OUR God, would not bring you this far to drop you now. Honey, I need to tell you about my vision last night," I said.

Stan looked at me puzzled, "What vision?"

I told him exactly what I saw while the song was playing. I then saw a sight I had not ever seen before. A beautiful sight that made me emotional once again.

I saw my husband tear up. The tears turned into crying and this might sound strange but at that moment my husband was the most handsome, most attractive man I had ever seen. Totally vulnerable. I could see his soul.

While the song was playing on my phone, I cupped my hands around his cheeks and said, "Stan, there is NOTHING you can do now but surrender your life into Jesus's hands."

"He loves you so much and He is going to carry you through, but it is all in His hands. Faith, that's what you need to have more than ever before. I KNOW you are going to be fine," I explained.

We both shed some tears and finished listening to the song. There was a peace that filled the room. It was now a time of living every second in total blind faith.

Just before 3 p.m. the nurse came to tell us that they should be fetching Stan to take him to the OR around 4 p.m. It sounded like a lifetime but with all the activity, the time flew by.

It was hard to control my thoughts as I kept thinking about the donor family. We were about to be connected on a level so few of us understand.

At 4:05 p.m. the porters arrived to take Stan to the OR. The nurse who was a little nervous all day, probably her first transplant recipient, quickly grabbed Stan's mask.

"Here, you have to wear this in the hallway to the OR," she said nervously and rushed to put it on as she also needed to make sure his heart monitor and other equipment were in place to leave the room.

She tried to put the mask on while she was already turning around, resulting in her putting the mask over Stan's eyes. She didn't even notice as she was already turned around working on the monitors.

Stan lay there for a second and I gently pulled the mask down off his eyes, over his mouth. He looked at me and we both started laughing. We didn't say anything to her. We just kept it between us at the moment.

The anesthesiologist arrived to walk with Stan and the team to the OR. It was time to say…what do you say? I was NOT going to allow the enemy to tell me this is "goodbye."

"You got this, God has got you," I said instead of goodbye.

I leaned over to kiss Stan.

"I love you so much, I'll see you in the morning, okay? I will see you with your new heart," I said.

"I love you too, honey," Stan said and I stood back for the porters to wheel the bed and all his accessories down the hallway to the OR.

The anesthetist touched my shoulder and said, "He is in good hands."

"Yes he is," I replied with a smile as I tried to hold back the tears.

Watching Stan being wheeled down the hallway was the most surreal feeling. I stood there till they took the turn at the end of the hallway, till I couldn't see them anymore.

I turned around and made my way to the elevators. I was flooded with emotion. I made it to the coffee shop and sat down at a table on the furthest end of the dining area.

I took a deep breath and messaged Stewart and the rest of the family.

"Please pray, Stan has just gone in for transplant surgery, could take anywhere from 8 to 16 hours depending on how things go, according to the doctors," I wrote to the family.

I didn't send a general update to friends as I wanted to have good news of a successful transplant.

Everyone was still under the impression he would have had the balloon pump moved that morning, not knowing the miracle that was busy unfolding.

I took a few deep breaths again and thanked God for the fact that I knew He was going to perform this miracle. It was already a miracle that Stan got a heart so soon.

Thirteen days after being listed. Having faith did not take the emotions and the stress away but it did give me a sense of peace. Indescribable peace.

I called my friend Thamar Jacobs in South Africa and we spoke for a while. Thamar has always been my wing woman and my sanity in times of chaos. It was the middle of the night for her but she made time as she wanted to know how I was coping.

We spoke for a little while and I went to get a cup of coffee. I knew there was no point sitting at the hospital but for some reason I need to be there, just a little bit longer.

At 5 p.m. my phone rang and I recognized the number as one of the hospital numbers.

"Hello?" I answered.

"Hi Mrs. Gregory, I just wanted to let you know we have the donor heart in hand and it looks really good. We are going to start surgery now and will call you once everything is done," a friendly voice explained.

"Thank you!" I said.

The recipient of a heart is not surgically touched until the team has the heart in hand, in the OR. The reason for this is that sometimes there is a physical issue with the heart and the team might decide not to go ahead with the surgery.

The recipient is then taken back to the room without any surgery. These situations are called "dry runs". Another blessing, Stan did not have a "dry run". This was it.

I prayed once more and asked the Lord to guide every person in that OR. To give everyone extraordinary ability, wisdom, energy, ability, and to guide each person. I prayed the Lord would be with Stan and bring him peace, and most importantly carry him through this miracle.

I bought dinner at the coffee shop and left for my temporary "home." I knew this was going to be a long night as I would not be able to sleep until I heard from the doctors.

Driving home I had that strange indescribable feeling again watching cars pass me, everyone totally oblivious to the fact that they were busy sawing open my husband's chest, cutting out his heart to put a new one in.

I visualized the donor family on their way home, just like me, but for them there was no more hope. Their loved one didn't make it, while my loved one was busy fighting for his life.

It is a weird reality. That reality of life and death happening and yet the world doesn't come to a standstill. Life continues.

I picked at the food when I got home and took a long warm bath before I laid down on the bed. It felt like I was in prayer all the time. I kept seeing Stan in the OR with his chest split open and his bed surrounded by doctors and nurses.

Stan was born in Mount Kisco, New York, not far from the hospital. Westchester Medical Center is in the town of Valhalla, NY. Valhalla, how ironic. The place Vikings believed they went to when they died.

At 5.45 p.m. my husband, the man I always called, "my Viking", died in the town of Valhalla, NY.

BUT GOD!

Ezekiel 36:26

I will give you a new heart and put a new spirit in you; I will remove from you your heart of stone and give you a heart of flesh.

My new husband, the Jesus Warrior, was about to be born as Dr. Kai continued stitching in the new heart.

At 8.30 p.m. my phone rang. It was once again one of the hospital numbers. Why are they calling? What happened? Is Stan ok?

It's only been 3.5 hours? Surgery would take more than six hours at least they said. This is too soon! So much flashed through my mind in that split second.

"Hello?" I answered frantically.

"Mrs. Gregory?" the male voice said.

"Yes?" I replied.

"Mrs. Gregory, this is Doctor Kai, I operated on your husband Stanley," he said.

Operated?? Past tense? Again so much flashed through my mind. It's been only three and a half hours. This CAN NOT be good news?

"Yes, Dr. Kai?" I said very nervously.

"I just called to let you know they are closing him up now," Dr. Kai said.

"What do you mean?" I interrupted.
Why were they closing him up? Did he die? Did something go wrong? My legs turned to jelly and I could feel my heart beating in my throat.

"They are closing his chest," Dr. Kai said, sounding a little confused at my question.

"Is he okay?" I asked.

"Yes, everything went well. The heart started beating immediately and very strong. There were no problems. He did well," Dr. Kai said.

"So everything is okay and all done?" I asked again.

Looking back I think Doctor Kai must have thought this lady is weird. She keeps asking if her husband is okay and he keeps telling me that it went well.

"Yes, he did well," Dr. Kai confirmed.

"Thank you, doctor. Thank you SO much," I said.

"You are welcome," Dr. Kai responded.

I couldn't believe it. It took 3.5 hours. 3.5 hours for a total heart transplant!

It took me a couple of minutes to come to the full realization that God pulled Stan through in record time! Miracle time!

God-smacked, I called Stewart and messaged everyone. I was in awe of God's goodness and just cried in gratitude.

I finally fell asleep late that night, praying Stan was not in pain or too uncomfortable.

"Thank you Papa. Thank you Jesus. Papa I am overflowing with gratitude. You have kept to Your promise. Thank you! Papa please continue to be with Stan. Allow him to heal as miraculously as well. You are my promise keeper.

Thank you that you will not allow him to have pain. Thank you for keeping him calm as he still has a breathing tube. Thank you for all the blessings Papa. Thank you!" I kept praying. I was in awe of God's goodness.

CHAPTER 8

Touched By An Angel

Thursday, December 2, 2021

I slept surprisingly well and woke up at 7 a.m. I called the Cardiac Thoracic ICU, also known as the CTICU, and asked the nurse how Stan was doing and if I could come to see him during visiting hours.

"Morning, Mrs. Gregory. Your husband is doing well. You are more than welcome to come to see him during visiting hours," the nurse said.

I was so relieved but I knew he had a long road of recovery ahead. There was now a new heart beating in his chest and new hope for a healthy life but a challenging time of healing.

Driving to the hospital I didn't know what to expect. I knew he might still have a breathing tube and just pictured the worst to brace myself to not be too shocked at what I would find.

I was early and had my morning coffee at the coffee shop. Sitting at that little round table the enemy tried to have a go at me. Messing with my mind and planting doubt.

I surrendered once more and said, "Lord, I know you are going to complete this miracle. Please remove the doubt. Please heal Stan's body and thank you for completing this miracle, Amen."

Within a few minutes, I received an email from an organization the transplant social worker, Bryan, told me about a couple of days earlier.

This incredible organization called, Harboring Hearts, is based in NYC and they help heart transplant recipients from out of town by providing various types of financial support.

I opened the email and I believe my mouth fell open.

"Dear Mrs. Gregory," the email started.

"We would like to send you grocery vouchers to the value of $600 and a coffee shop voucher at the hospital for $100." I was blown away. A total of $700!

Not only was this a HUGE financial help as everything closer to NYC was so much more expensive than it was back home but the number *seven* has always been the number I associated with the presence of God. It was God's number.

God was sending me a sign reassuring me He is ALWAYS in total control and He intends to finish the promise of a miracle.

The promise He made weeks earlier when I stood in my kitchen back home.

"I am going to perform a miracle in Stan's life, I am not done with him yet."

He is in control. I needed to let go of the doubt. God knows our hearts and he knows mine. I needed even more reassurance and my Papa was about to give me that reassurance. He was about to drown me in confirmations.

The email from Harboring Hearts continued by saying they are also able to assist with accommodation costs while I was down in the city. What a miracle in itself.

Harboring Hearts was a blessing to us in a time we needed support most. They took the stress out of my life so I could fully focus on supporting Stan. They continued to be a blessing for months after the surgery.

I was sitting there watching people go about their business and I wanted to get up and yell, GOD IS SO GOOD!

I put my hand up into the air and just said. "Thank you, Jesus!"

My phone rang. It was my friend from back home, Kim Michielson. Kim has always been an angel in my life and helping people in crisis just comes naturally to her.

She started and was managing a GoFundMe account for Stan and I.

"Hey, Kimmy!" I answered.

"Honey, have you checked your GoFundMe?" she said.

"No? Why?" I asked.

"Someone has just deposited $777 into the account and another person deposited $77," she said excitedly.

"What??" I said.

Kim had no idea about the Harboring Hearts gift or that 7 was a special number to me, especially at that moment.

When I explained that Harboring Hearts just sent me $700 of vouchers she almost started crying with me!

God was flooding me with confirmation and reassurance that He intended to finish this miracle with Stan. "***I am not done with Stan yet,***" I heard God saying again.

It was finally time for visiting hours. I was nervous. Nervous about seeing Stan. Not knowing what to expect and being an empath makes it even tougher to see someone in pain or discomfort.

As I stood in the lobby, at the elevator, I had a supernatural experience.

It was strange to me that there were so few people waiting for the elevators. Normally it was buzzing with people at the start of visiting hours. There were three elevators, all next to each other on one side of the lobby.

I stood in front of the middle elevator, leaving enough space for people who might be getting out on this floor when the elevator arrived.

A lady, whom I am CONVINCED was an Angel, stood a few steps behind me.

I felt a tap on my shoulder and I looked back at her. I cannot describe what she looked like except she was smiling and there was an Angelic feeling beaming off of her.

She smiled and said, "Look, that's a perfect number," as she pointed to the top of the elevators.

I turned and looked back to the elevators and saw the numbers above each elevator showing which floor the elevator was currently on.

7 7 7

"Are you KIDDING me? What?" I said as I turned back to the Angel, my mouth literally hanging open in surprise.

She had a huge smile on her face like she KNEW what the number meant to me.

"You have no idea what that number means to me," I said.

"Oh I do, it is a GREAT number," she replied with a smile and pointed back at the middle elevator as it arrived on the floor.

I was covered in goosebumps from the top of my head to the tips of my toes.

I got into the elevator and pressed the second-floor button, completely God-smacked at what just happened.

As the elevator doors closed I saw the Angel, just standing there, smiling. She didn't move. She never got into the elevator.

There are no words to describe what I was feeling. There was NO doubt in my mind, I was just touched by an Angel!

I got off on the fourth floor and walked towards the CTICU.

I KNEW Stan was going to be just fine as God was showing me so many confirmations all within minutes of each other. The excitement I felt was indescribable. My Papa sent me an ANGEL!!!

He chose ME, little old me, to send an Angel of confirmation. I am a Child of God!

I called the front desk from the waiting room to check if I could come through the security doors to see Stan.

"Certainly Mrs. Gregory. The nurse is with him but you can come through," the friendly voice said.

As I walked up to the front desk I was greeted by the same voice.

"Good morning, Mrs. Gregory, you can go through and see your husband, the nurse is with him. He is in room 7," she said.

"Room 7? Did you say room 7?" I asked.

"Yes, right at the end of the hallway on the right," she replied.

I started laughing. She must have wondered why but I was too excited to get to Stan and there was no time to explain.

Besides, I was speechless by God's continuous confirmation. He put my husband in room 7!

Now I knew WITHOUT a doubt Stan was IN God's hands.

I opened the room door and a nurse looked up at me.

"You must be Mrs. Gregory?" she asked.

"Morning, yes. How is my husband?" I asked.

Stan had his eyes open and he was clearly alert but still had a breathing tube. I quickly scanned the room. I saw so many extra machines, and lines and was surprised to see the balloon pump still there too.

I walked up to Stan and said, "Hey handsome, you got a new heart! Don't try to speak, ok? Everyone says you are doing so well."

He smiled and blinked.

Later Stan would tell me he didn't even remember getting the surgery. The whole transplant day was a blur to him.

As I leaned closer to him he started blinking more as if he was trying to say something. Maybe it was because we knew each other so well or maybe it's my super empathetic side but I knew what he was trying to say.

"Do you want me to wipe your eyes?" I asked.

He blinked and nodded slightly. The nurse passed me a packet of wet wipes and I wiped his eyes. I wiped his forehead and the rest of his face that wasn't covered in tubes or wires.

I kept reassuring him he was doing well. Doctor Levine walked into the room.

"Good morning," he said excitedly.

"Good morning doctor," I replied.

"Stan is doing exceptionally well. There is going to be a lot happening today but I could not be more pleased with how he is doing," Dr. Levine said.

"Why does he still have the balloon pump?" I asked.

"We are helping the new heart ease into the new body as gently as possible with as much support as possible. We will be removing the balloon pump this morning. You will also notice he is on a pacemaker which is why he has a steady heartbeat.

We will slowly drop the support and allow the heart to do more work over the next few days. The breathing tube will also come out later today when his levels are where he will be comfortable without the tube," he explained.

"Thank you doctor. Thank you!" I said. I was overflowing with gratitude.

"You're welcome. I will be in and out all day checking on him so please feel free to ask any questions at any time. Remember, you, me, and Stan are now in a relationship for the next 20+ years. We are going to be seeing a lot of each other and speak regularly," he assured me.

I found such comfort in those words. Dr. Levine has a tone, a confidence and a mannerism that always reassures you. Even if it is not great news, he delivers it so well that you don't even worry.

"Thank you!" I replied.

When the doctor left the room I asked the nurse if Stan was getting anything for pain.

"No, not at the moment," she replied.

"WHAT?" I almost choked on my spit.

"Nothing for pain?" I said.

"We have liquid Tylenol if he needs it. She leaned over to Stan and asked, "Mr. Gregory are you in any pain?"

Stan looked over at her and moved his head from side to side slowly indicating "no".

How is this even possible? They cracked open his chest, took out his old heart, put a new one in and he has NO pain? My warrior husband once again proved just how strong he was.

Stan looked over at me. He found it hard to even just lift his hand off the bed. His whole body was swollen and I didn't think it strange after what he had just been through.

It wasn't just the heart that needed to gently be eased into the new body but the body that needed to accept the new heart.

"What is it honey?" I asked.

He lifted his one hand a few inches off the bed and pointed to the window into the hallway.

"I don't understand honey, what do you want me to do?" I asked.

He pointed to the window again and managed to lift his other hand off the bed too.

With two pointed fingers towards the hallway, he pulled his fingers closer to each other.

I got a glimpse of the nurse staring at him confused and it was like we were all playing a game of Charades. She was about to run to find their alphabet indicator so he could spell it out when it hit me.

I shouted out like I would if we did play a game of charades.

"You want me to close the curtains??" I shouted.

Stan nodded excitedly that I understood, smiling.

"And you want me to switch the lights off too right?" I added and he smiled bigger, nodding yes once again.

The nurse sighed in relief that I understood and quickly started drawing the curtains and turned to dim the lights.

"Wow, I am glad you are here Mrs. Gregory, I would never have understood that. Please stay till we remove the breathing tube," she laughed.

Stan smiled.

"I am not going anywhere," I said and sat down next to Stan as I took his hand. His hand was swollen and I struggled to get my fingers between his.

"Sleep honey, I am right here. You need rest. You are ok. Everyone is saying how well you are doing so just rest," I said and he blinked and closed his eyes.

There was a small opening between the now drawn curtains looking into the hallway and I could see people constantly moving back and forth. The ICU was always busy.

The nurse was in the room with us all the time checking his blood pressure and all the monitors.

I sat staring at the heart monitor. Constant heartbeats due to the pacemaker. It was the most surreal feeling knowing that less than 24 hours ago Stan's old heart was struggling to beat in his chest and now someone else's heart is beating so strong inside of him.

These are things we never think about. We never think transplant will affect us personally until we get there and it becomes a part of our life.

Strange thoughts crossed my mind as I was sitting there. I grew up only a few minutes from Groote Schuur Hospital in Cape Town, South Africa where Dr. Christiaan Barnard did the very first successful human to human heart transplant in 1967.

One of my father's friends, Dr. Cecyl Moss, was one of the doctors on that team. My dad only told me this when Stan received a heart.

Here I was, sitting in Westchester Medical Center in New York, USA next to my husband in 2021 who just became the recipient of a donor's heart.

Stan's blood pressure was monitored very closely among many other things. It was crucial to keep his blood pressure under a certain level to ensure the heart is not put under unnecessary pressure. I was fascinated with the medical information about transplants. How things have changed since 1967.

I imagined Dr. Barnard, if he could be there in the room with us right then. I could imagine his voice would pitch higher and higher as it did when he became excited speaking about heart transplants.

A few hours later three doctors came in saying they wanted to remove the balloon pump from Stan's groin and it would take about an hour so I decided to go and have a coffee break.

The room was small and seeing as it was a medical procedure they needed me to leave while they did the removal.

I used the time to update family and friends including Candy and Karen. They were over the moon with joy hearing Stan received a heart and that he was doing well. Karen could not wait to share the news with Dave who kept improving in the ICU.

It was good to walk back into Stan's room and see more space available. The balloon pump was gone and the big brace-like support was off his leg.

The nurse pulled up a chair and I sat down next to Stan. I took his hand again. He started hiccupping and it became so violent that his shoulder would lift off the bed every time with each hiccup.

I became anxious as I knew this must cause some pain with his whole body moving with every hiccup.

"Are you ok Honey? Do you maybe want some Tylenol for pain? Maybe it will help relax you a little," I asked Stan.

He turned his head slightly towards me and nodded, "yes" while blinking his eyes.

The nurse leaned over and asked for confirmation that he would like Tylenol. He nodded yes again. She put a Tylenol IV on and within five minutes I could see Stan relaxing more and finally the hiccups stopped. He fell asleep again and I felt like I could breathe easier too.

A specialist doctor came in to check his oxygen levels and kept drawing blood to see if they could remove the breathing tube.

"He is doing well, I think early this evening we will be able to remove the tube," he reassured me.

Stan had a central line in his neck. It is a catheter placed into the jugular vein. This made it so much easier for the constant blood draws to check and monitor levels.

This way they didn't have to poke him every time. I called it "blood on tap" which the nurses found hilarious.

I truly have nothing but good to say about the staff in the Intensive Care Units. They were all incredible.

I kept taking breaks away from Stan that day because I felt he tried to stay awake if I was there. If I broke away for an hour at a time he would sleep.

I made sure I was there enough to reassure him that I am around and that he simply needs to focus on sleeping as much as he could.

Around 6 p.m. I decided to call it a day as they were planning to remove the breathing tube and then do a shift change which meant I would have to step out of the room anyway.

I said bye to Stan and he looked at peace about me going. I reassured him I would be there at 11 a.m. the following morning.

I also made sure he understood that I would check in with the nurse later in the evening and make sure he is okay.

I walked out of the hospital on a spiritual high. I would call it a spiritual hangover. It was a busy day filled with emotion and miracles. A lot of action around Stan medically but he was doing well and I was overflowing with gratitude.

Friday, December 3, 2021

When I walked into room 7 in the CTICU on Friday, December 3rd, I was greeted by the most handsome man with a smile to die for.

Stan looked incredible. He looked 15 years younger, awake, alert, and like a completely different person.

"Oh my word, you look incredible!" I said and walked over to kiss him.

"Morning honey," he replied with a big smile.

"He got up and sat in the chair earlier this morning for his breakfast," the nurse said enthusiastically.

"What?? You have been UP?" I was shocked.

"Yes. He did very well," the nurse replied.

I was so surprised that he was up so soon after the transplant and especially after he has not been on his feet for more than three weeks.

"Wow Stan, I am super proud of you, that's incredible," I said.

Stan smiled like a little kid who just got praised for doing a good job. What an achievement.

They set his heartbeat down to fewer beats per minute as they explained they would. It went from 120 beats to 110 beats. This would continue till they would switch off the pacemaker completely allowing the heart to work on its own and then remove it.

Dr. Levine came in and explained how happy he was with Stan's progress and how well he is doing. I was blown away by how quickly my husband was bouncing back. They explained that if he continued the way he was he would be out of ICU in a few days.

Wow. Three days ago we were waiting on a balloon pump to be moved and here we are, Stan has a new heart and is healing at one incredible speed. But that's my husband. He seems to hit things hard but bounces back every time.

I took a photo of Stan as I could not get over how incredibly handsome he looked and as much as he hated to have his photo taken he even smiled for the photo.

Our day was spent getting him comfortable and moving into the chair for each meal. He needed to move as much as possible to prevent blood clots and also for his general recovery. After each "move" he would be tired but a quick snooze fixed it every time.

I kept staring at him. It was a miracle that he was alive and got a heart only thirteen days after being listed.

I belonged to a group on Facebook for Families of Heart Transplant patients and I saw a post of a young guy who was waiting on a heart and mentioned he was now on day 87 of waiting in hospital.

This was a miracle indeed and we were flooded with God's favor.

Stan's meals were still only broths and jellies but his appetite increased and he started asking for double servings.

I was too happy to go ask the nurse for another meal as it indicated healing was happening in Stan's body. Later he was treated with yogurt, his favorite.

Stan had developed steroid-induced diabetes due to the Prednisone medication. He was on 35mg but this would be dropped by 5mg every time they did a biopsy indicating there is no rejection.

Once he is off the steroid he would hopefully not need to take insulin anymore.

At this time everything possible was done medically to support the heart to adapt to the new body and for the body to accept this new heart.

I spent a lot of time between nurses and doctors poking at him massaging his feet.

His feet were still swollen from the surgery and hurting a little as he hadn't been on his feet for weeks except for getting up to sit in the chair.

Stewart called me as I was heading "home" and said he was going to come to see Stan on Sunday and stay over the night and see him again Monday.

I checked with the owner of the guesthouse and she was kind enough to prepare another bedroom for Stewart. Another blessing.

CHAPTER 9

Delirium

Saturday, December 4, 2021

I found Stan sitting in the chair next to the bed having yogurt when I got to his room. It quickly became clear there was a lot of confusion again and it was disturbing even though I was warned about ICU delirium and I had witnessed some of it before.

The nurse asked me shortly after I walked into the room, "Mrs. Gregory, do you by any chance know where your husband's cell phone is? He was saying we lost the phone this morning."

I could sense a little frustration from her side, understandably so as no-one likes to be accused of something they didn't do.

"I have it right here in my bag. Dr. Levine told me to take all his belongings on the day of the transplant as he was going to be moved to a different unit after and he would not be able to use a phone for the first few days anyway," I said.

I looked over to Stan and said, "They didn't lose it honey, I got it and if you want to keep it here today you can, I have your charger too."

It was frustrating having to deal with a stranger again. During the morning I saw that he was fighting sleep while I was in the room.

At 2 p.m. I told him I was going to take a break and go to the store to get a few things. I reasoned that maybe this way he will sleep while I am gone.

That's exactly what he did when I went to do some retail therapy in the town he was born in. Mount Kisco.

It was once again a sense of loneliness that hit me while driving. It would have been so wonderful to see these places with Stan.

Even though I was relieved about my husband doing well I was sad that I did sightseeing by myself. Even if it was limited to a drive to the store.

When I got back to the hospital, I ran into Dr. Lanier in the hallway. The doctor who gave me the reality gut punch that Stan would have to go to hospice if he didn't get onto the transplant list.

"Hi Dr. Lanier," I said as he walked toward me.

"Hi there. Your husband is doing exceptionally well," he said.

"Doc, it's a miracle. I am so grateful," I replied.

"Absolutely. I don't believe your husband would have lived past the end of December if he didn't get a heart, I am truly happy for you both," he said.

"Thank you so much Doctor, I am so grateful to you all," I said.

"You are so welcome," he replied.

As I continued walking to Stan's unit the reality of the miracle hit me once again. I could be sitting at my husband's bedside at hospice watching him die, but here we are.

Stan has a new heart. He is doing great and he is on the road to recovery.

Stan was sleeping when I got to his room but soon woke up. I massaged his feet a little again and put some special lotion on that I had bought to moisturize his super dry feet.

"I am excited about Stew visiting tomorrow," he said.

Ten or so minutes later he would ask me when Stew is planning to visit him again. The confusion and memory loss was disturbing to me again but I knew it was considered "normal."

For the remainder of the afternoon Stan kept fighting the sleep so I decided to call it a day and also needed to get some laundry done at the house. Up to this point I have been handwashing a few items and was relieved people were wearing masks because I felt like I was starting to smell.

It was the greatest, freshest feeling having all my laundry done later that evening. I took a long warm bath and made myself a small dinner. I was mentally exhausted. It is a type of exhaustion that is hard to put into words.

Sunday, December 5, 2021

If I thought Stan was confused the day before I didn't know what was awaiting me when I arrived at the hospital.

Stan was about to prove that hospital delirium is a VERY real thing but knowing Stan he had to make it special, in a funny kind of way.

As I walked into his room he seemed concerned.

"What's wrong honey?" I asked.

"I am NOT very happy," he said.

"Why? What's happening?' I asked again.

"Why is the guy across the hallway allowed to bring his boat into the hospital?" Stan asked.

I bolted to the drawn curtain to see what was going on across from Stan's room.

"Do you see? That's not fair!" Stan said.

I obviously didn't see a boat but I knew to climb into his world as it would not escalate his frustration.

"I agree honey, that's not ok," I said and drew the curtain closed as I turned back to Stan.

"You need to take this up with management, Liesl. Please, this is not ok," Stan insisted.

"Most definitely, I will do that when I go downstairs for coffee later," I assured him.

He seemed to accept my suggestion and left it at that. For now.

I distracted him with his chocolate-flavored muscle milk and his yogurt. It worked. At least for five minutes.

The nurse came in to check on Stan and left the door ajar as she walked out. Stan could see another patient diagonally across from him and his eyes grew bigger and bigger.

With his jaw literally dropping, he shouted loudly and very seriously, "LIESL!"

"What?" I asked concerned as he startled me.

"Did you see that guy in the bed across there?" he asked, pulling me closer by my arm.

"Yes, I did, why?" I responded.

With a look of total shock, panic, concern and almost disgust, Stan said, "I hope I didn't get that guy's heart, he's OLD!"

I started laughing.

"Why are you laughing Liesl, this is serious!" Stan said.

I laughed, even more, I simply couldn't help laughing.

"Honey!" I said.

"What?" Stan replied.

"You did not get his heart," I said, and before I could finish Stan put his hand on his chest and gave a big "PHEW" with a sigh of relief.

He looked at me concerned again.

"Are you SURE?" he asked.

Trying not to laugh I replied, "I am positive! The person who left you their heart passed away, honey. You can't live without a heart. Your donor died," I explained.

Stan had a moment of sadness in his eyes when I said his donor died.

"It's ok," I said and gently touched his shoulder.

He lit up a little and his sadness turned back to relief.

Again he said, "That guy is OLD."

Moments like these I will never forget. I knew it was a temporary confusion so I tried not to get upset and allowed myself to laugh a little.

He kept peeking out the door staring at the man across the hallway like a little child that could not let go of something.

I kept trying to distract Stan with things when he started speaking no sense. I kept telling him Stewart was on his way and would visit him the next morning.

When Stan finally fell asleep I thought of the donor family again. I wondered if they have had a memorial or funeral for him or her. I sent prayers for peace to them. I had no idea how this person could have died but knew that this must be a devastating time for the family.

In the middle of the day I left for the store to find Stan an MP3 player. The ICU was so noisy day and night. It never stopped.

I thought if I could get Stan to listen to music with headphones he might sleep better.

When I returned to the hospital he just woke up and was much more lucid than earlier in the day. Thank God!

Stewart arrived later that evening and we spent some time catching up. We decided to get a few things done before we left for the hospital the next morning.

Monday, December 6, 2021

Stewart and I went to get some groceries early in the morning and headed to the hospital. Stan was a little confused but happy to see Stew and they immediately started their bantering again.

"Can I turn this button?" Stew asked, pretending he was going to turn Stan's pacemaker up.

"You want me to pull the fire alarm don't you?" Stan replied.

It was good to see Stan laughing a little.

Dr. Levine walked in and was glad to see Stan had another visitor.

"Stan is doing exceptionally well," Dr. Levine said.

"I am so grateful doc, thank you!" I replied. "Doc, is the confusion still normal?" I asked for reassurance.

"Oh definitely. It will get better when he moves out of ICU later this week. I am not worried about that at all," Dr. Levine explained.

He had a manner that always put your mind at ease but I also knew he is not the type of doctor who would hide information to spare you. He had a way of telling you facts, good or bad but left you feeling everything is under control.

"That is a relief," I said.

"Stan was bragging about you yesterday." Dr. Levine said.

"Why? What did he say?" I asked.

"Oh just about you pulling trucks and airplanes, nothing major," Dr. Levine laughed.

"Oh gosh yeah that was in my strongwoman years," I laughed.

"Impressive!" Dr. Levine said as he started heading out the door. "We will see you later but rest assured I am very happy with Stan's progress," he said before he left the room.

After Dr. Levine left Stan looked at me and said, "Liesl, you won't believe what they are doing across in the other room now. They started building the guy a boat launch!" Stan said disgustedly.

Stew looked at me with total confusion as to what that even meant. "I am sure it will stop today honey, I will speak to management again later," I replied and the confusion on Stewart's face got even more hilarious.

"Stew," I said, "Stan told me the guy across the hall brought his boat in, and I mean what kind of a hospital allows that?"

Stew realized this was part of Stan's delirium. I told him about it and replied, "So unfair!"

Stan and Stew continued bantering and nurses and doctors kept coming in and out of his room. It was truly amazing to see Stan returning to the man I knew while he was kidding around with Stew.

One of the things that made me fall in love with Stan originally was his humor. Sadly a lot of the humor faded over the past few years as he grew sicker.

When we left later in the evening the receptionist from CTICU, Stephanie, was at the front desk.

"Have a good night, Mrs. Gregory," she said as I walked past.

"Thank you and you too!" I replied.

"You are so nice. Seriously. You are one of the nicest people I have met," she continued.

"Aw thank you, Stephanie, I am sure you see a lot of people at their worst," I replied.

"Oh yes but you sure are a nice lady," she said again.

I wanted to hug her, what a sweet soul.

Stew and I were just about to leave the car park when my phone rang. It was Stan.

"Stan? Are you ok?" I answered.

"Yes, I am fine. Am I on speaker phone? Is Stew with you?" Stan asked.

"Yes. Why?" I replied.

"I wanted to tell you guys I just had a massive poo," Stan said.

We all burst out laughing.

"Good job honey, is that why you called?" I laughed.

"Yes, got to go, the nurse is going to clean me now," he laughed as he hung up.

Stewart and I looked at each other and had a good laugh at the Stan we knew so well. The old Stan slowly filtering through the confusion.

Tuesday, December 7, 2021

Stewart decided to join me at the hospital later as he would head back to North Carolina directly from the hospital later in the afternoon.

I was early having my usual coffee at my usual table at the hospital coffee shop. It struck me how many police officers started to gather at the front desk, and reception area.

My curiosity got the better of me and I walked over to two NYPD officers having coffee.

"Good morning, do you mind me asking why there are so many police officers here this morning?" I asked.

"Good morning!" the one officer replied with a smile. "We are here to show our support to a fellow officer," he said.

"He is being released today. He is a state trooper who got hit by a car a few days ago so we just came to do our thing and show him our support as he is released," the other officer explained.

"That is amazing and I am happy to hear he is being released. Thank you to all of you for your incredible service," I said.

"Thank you so much, you are welcome," they both replied.

While I waited for the visiting hours to start I was amazed at the fact that there were just more and more officers arriving. Soon the hospital staff also started gathering.

The officers then lined the hospital hallway from the injured officers' room to the front exit where an ambulance was awaiting to transport him home.

I could hear people clapping hands all the way down the hallway as they approached the front lobby. Everyone clapped and cheered while some hospital staff held up posters. "You did it." "Well done." It was heartwarming to see the support.

I noticed a young lady standing next to me who was also very excited. I had noticed her at the patient liaison desk at reception a few times before.

She looked at me and said, "This is always so good to see when they get to go home."

"It is amazing," I replied.

"I have seen you here for a few days now," she said.

"Oh yes, I have been visiting my husband since November 15th. He received a heart transplant on December 1st," I said.

"Oh wow. How is he doing?" she asked sincerely.

"Excellent, we are so grateful. Everything happened so quickly. I even forgot his bag of clothes rushing to get to the hospital so I guess I need to go do some shopping. Everything happened so quickly," I laughed.

"Are you from out of town?" she asked.

"Yes, we are from about six hours away, near Rochester," I replied.

"NO NO NO, You are not going to go buy stuff," she said as she grabbed my arm and started pulling me towards her office. "I have everything you might need," she said.

"What? Are you serious?" I asked.

"Yes! We have so much stuff for patients like your husband. Please come with me," she said as she dragged me into her office.

She opened a closet with drawers and asked, "What size does he wear?"

"Probably an extra-large right now," I said.

"Here, I got this," she said excitedly and started pulling brand new tracksuits, socks, T-shirts, and even toiletries out of the drawers.

"No need to go buy anything," she said and turned around to me to see why I was not responding.

I was in tears. I was dumbstruck by God's goodness. God-smacked again. His goodness was chasing after us in so many ways.

From this day I called that emotion "God-smacked" not gob smacked. God blew my breath away. Again. And again!

"Oh, don't cry honey," she said and walked over to me as she placed everything on a desk next to me.

She opened her arms inviting me for a hug and I embraced her in total gratitude.

"God has been so good supplying our EVERY need in this time and here you are being yet another angel in our lives," I cried.

"Aww don't cry. We are here to help where we can," she said and excitedly turned around to get even more things out of the closet.

I left that office with bags of clothes and toiletries for Stan.

I couldn't wait to get to Stan to tell him about yet another miracle. He looked good and the confusion seemed a little less. Stewart joined us for a while before heading back to North Carolina.

It meant the world to Stan to see his brother during this time.

Later the day they removed Stan's central line and the doctor said I could stay in the room if I wasn't squeamish.

"Me? Oh, doc if you only knew the stuff I have witnessed. I will be fine," I assured him.

I was shocked at how thick the line was. He continued to put pressure on the spot for 5 minutes after he pulled the line which was uncomfortable for Stan but Nurse Sebastian quickly came to the rescue with some Tylenol.

It was another big step forward as Stan felt more free having less equipment attached to him and no longer had the line pulling at his neck every time he moved.

Stan became confused again later in the day. Restless. It exhausted me. "Pull the curtain. Open the curtain. Switch on the light. Switch off the light. Help me sit up. Help me lay down. Help me get up," he said over and over.

Nothing I seemed to do was right. When dinner arrived and I lifted the cover from the plate and he saw the fish he said, "I'm not eating that."

Stan had again become a stranger and even though I knew it was normal, I struggled to cope with these moments.

I decided it was better to break for a coffee and get some space. The nurse said he would order Stan some chicken and told me to take my time.

While having coffee, watching doctors, nurses, and visitors coming and going, I had a call from Elaine Valencia, one of Stan's heart team Nurse Practitioners.

She was super compassionate and became a lifeline in the coming months. Always available and willing to help. She also seemed to understand Stan's type of humor and his personality.

"Hi Liesl, are you somewhere near the hospital?" she asked.

"Yes, I am downstairs having a coffee break. Is Stan okay?" I asked.

"Everything is fine. I just needed you to sign the consent form for Stan for his first biopsy Thursday. He is so full of wiring and said you should sign if you can?" she explained.

"Absolutely. I will be back with Stan in about 10 minutes," I said.

"Perfect. I will meet you in his room then I can explain the procedure to you both," she said.

The biopsies would be weekly during the first month, then bimonthly, and then monthly until six months. IF it all looked good we could start what is called Blood-mapping which is a blood test to check for possible rejection.

I met Elaine back in Stan's room and signed the paperwork. They were planning to move Stan out of ICU the next day.

Everything was happening so quickly. One week in ICU after a transplant. It became clear the doctors were not just being nice when they said he was doing exceptionally well. This truly was a miracle.

Zaan and Taylor were also arriving in a couple of days to visit Stan and again the guest house owner was such a blessing in allowing them to stay in the second bedroom. That house became our home during this time.

This experience was starting to give completely new meaning to, "Home is where the heart is".

CHAPTER 10

Healing

Wednesday, December 8, 2021 – One week after the transplant

Stan had less and less confusion. Thank God. I struggled to deal with the stranger my husband became on and off the past couple of weeks.

Stan was transferred from the ICU to a recovery floor after I got all his things packed. They moved him to room 403. Yup, a 7 again. 4+0+3=7. God was walking this journey right beside us. Finishing this miracle.

Stan had his biopsy the following morning. No rejection and his numbers looked excellent according to Dr. Levine. His loop recorder from the old heart was removed from his chest, just under the skin, in a small procedure leaving yet another scar on his chest.

One thing Stan has never worried about was his scars. They were his battle reminders. Each tells a story.

The following days were filled with Stan getting stronger. Walking to the bathroom. Stronger each day.

Zaan and Taylor visited for a couple of days and it was not just energizing for me to see them but for Stan to see them, as well.

During this time they also got to meet Candy and Karen at the hospital and they were shocked to realize how close they live to each other.

Karen shared that Dave was slowly still getting stronger and he was a fighter without a doubt. I got excited at the prospect of having a summer BBQ when Stan and Dave would be all healed up and for them to meet.

Karen excitedly said, "I told Dave about Stan's transplant and he almost became emotional. He was so excited about the journey for Stan and the miracle of life. It really inspired him." This was so heartwarming to hear.

During Stan's stay in the hospital, I also got to meet Dave Gray, one of the hospital's patient advocates. No, Dave is much more than just an advocate. Dave is a counselor to many patients who are waiting on a donor heart. He has been a support to families and even families of donors.

Dave received a transplant at Westchester six years ago.

It was a blessing to be able to speak to him when we needed to even though it was on video calls due to the limitations of the COVID regulations.

I mentioned to Dave that it was tough not knowing much about the donor. All we knew was the person was younger than 50 years old.

Dave recommended we contact LiveOnNY. This organ procurement organization would have more on the donor if the donor was from NY.

We decided to wait until we were back at home in Lakeville before we reached out to them. It seemed too soon and I wanted to respect their privacy during their time of grief.

Tuesday, December 14, 2021

Stan was supposed to be transferred to the rehabilitation unit right next door to the hospital the past Sunday but again, due to COVID and tremendous staff shortages the transfer ambulance kept being postponed.

They finally arrived at 2 a.m. on Tuesday which annoyed me as I was not happy for Stan to be moved out in the cold night when he has a suppressed immune system but he had to take the opportunity or miss it for a few more days.

Stan was desperate to get out of the hospital setting. He settled in at rehab with a really comfortable room, His own little bar fridge and enough space to move.

He had a private room and had a lovely big window overlooking a garden and it felt more and more like home. A far way from the CICIU with a smallish room, no outside window, and constant lights and people moving around.

Even though it was comfortable Stan was wanting to get out of the hospital setting completely.

Rehab was needed though and here he would become even stronger with the help of physiotherapists helping him with confidence in climbing stairs and doing basic chores daily.

The few weeks of laying down and then the big surgery took a knock on his strength but Stan was adamant to work hard and gain the strength back.

Stan was still in a daily routine of physical therapy twice a day as well as other therapies to help him strengthen. It exhausted him at first but this allowed him to sleep a little better as he became physically tired.

It did feel more like being out of the hospital by being able to wear his own clothes and the setup was more personal.

But it wasn't home. Stan became more eager to join me at the guest house.

We decided to stay in the city till his biopsies became a two-week thing as a weekly trip would simply be too tough on him and just too much driving.

Besides, I had the place booked till January 8th, so we did not need to rush home straight away.

He worked hard every day to be able to go home as soon as possible. It became his motivation. If he was able to climb the flight of stairs he would be able to leave.

The transplant team would come see him every day to see his progress and speak to him about a possible discharged date. At this time they were planning on around December 27th.

Stan could not bear being there for that long and asked Dr. Levine if he could be discharged earlier as we would still be in the area for a few more weeks.

Dr. Levine was happy for Stan to leave once he was able to climb stairs comfortably and once all his medication had arrived which we would be taking home with us.

Once I had the medication education from the transplant team, we would be all set to be discharged.

CHAPTER 11

A Christmas Miracle

Tuesday, December 21, 2021

We got our Christmas Miracle and Stan's discharge date finally arrived, a little earlier than expected.

It felt like months had passed and that maybe, just maybe, our roller coaster was finally in the straight run before it would stop.

I made sure I stocked up on groceries before Stan came home as Christmas was drawing near and stores were becoming crowded. I also tried to stay away from large crowds at this point as I didn't want to be a carrier of something that could affect Stan with his suppressed immune system.

Stan's amount of medication was overwhelming to me at first but the team made it much easier with their printouts and education session.

We decided I would do the medications as I just wanted Stan to focus all his energy on healing and details was not his forte.

I got a large file with information as well as a blood pressure machine, a glucose machine, and a bag of medication.

Finally, it was time. 42 days in total from the day I dropped him off at the ED at Rochester General Hospital to this day when he was being discharged at Westchester Medical Center.

Forty-two days. During this time Stan was airlifted, received a total of three balloon pumps, and an Impella heart pump, diagnosed with COVID, quarantined for fourteen days, had a brain bleed and a small stroke, got listed for a heart transplant, and received a heart transplant and a loop recorder removed and recovered from all of these events and procedures.

Stan got into the wheelchair, greeted everyone for the last time, and was wheeled out the double doors to the car.

When we arrived at the guest house Stan settled in and I got into the medication ritual. It was good to be able to lay next to my husband again. Putting my hand on his chest as I did on the morning of November 9, 2021.

But this time, his heart was beating strongly. I laid there thanking God for his donor and this second chance at life.

We returned to the hospital two days later for Stan's weekly biopsy and again, no rejection. God was finishing this miracle. Just as He promised.

I wanted to make it a special Christmas even though we would not be able to see the kids but Stan had no idea there was a surprise planned for him. Stewart and his wife Amy decided to come and spend Christmas with us in our little temporary Yonkers, NY home.

Late in the afternoon of Christmas Eve, Stew and Amy arrived. Stan could not believe his eyes when they walked into the room.

"Now I understand why you got so much food for tomorrow," Stan laughed. "There is no way that could be for just two people," he said.

I was overwhelmed with gratitude as we sat in the lounge that evening. A massive Christmas tree with beautiful lights next to the fireplace. Surrounded by family. A blessed Christmas Eve. My husband is alive and well, next to me.

"I could have been sitting next to your bed in hospice right now, holding your hand as you were dying," I said softly to Stan and I could feel the tears surfacing.

"I know," Stan replied and put his hand out for me to hold while fighting back tears himself.

I thought of the donor's family. How unbelievably difficult this Christmas must be for them.

"Jesus, please comfort them. Hold each family member in Your hands please Papa," I prayed softly.

We had a wonderful Christmas day with Stew and Amy. Delicious lunch and Christmas movies while we all relaxed and laughed, enjoying and celebrating the birth of Jesus and celebrating LIFE!

Stan and I became a little homesick over the next few days after Stew and Amy left again and wanted to head back to Lakeville, our real home.

We decided that after Stan's biopsy on December 30th we would head back home and return two weeks later for the next biopsy rather than spend another two weeks occupying ourselves in the guest house.

We felt we needed to start the New Year at home.

We both went to have a COVID test done the Tuesday morning so we would have results for Stan's procedure by Thursday, but by now the news had created chaos in the city by saying if you have a runny nose or are sneezing you probably have COVID.

Suddenly there were National Guard directing vehicles at the test station and lines which took almost an hour to get through.

By Thursday morning we still didn't have any results but the amazing Dr. Levine came to the rescue with a plan.

"We will simply treat Stan like he is COVID positive and follow the protocols. We will take you to a different unit but we will make it work," he explained.

Dr. Levine, the problem solver to the rescue once more. I believe he wears a superman shirt under his white coat, or maybe this Angel folds away his wings.

By the time we arrived at the hospital on Thursday morning, Stan mentioned he had a little bit of a runny nose. Dr. Levine suggested having a COVID test done on Stan so they could eliminate that he was actually positive. Just in case.

The biopsy was once again negative and Dr. Levine mentioned how good Stan's numbers looked. We headed to the guest house to start packing as we wanted to leave for home the following morning.

Around 4 p.m. my phone rang.

"Hi, Liesl, this is Dr. Levine. We got Stan's COVID test back and he tested positive. Where are you guys now?" he asked.

"Oh no! We are still in Yonkers, Doc. We wanted to leave early tomorrow morning," I said.

"Ok, I suggest you bring Stan for an antibody infusion before you head back. I will arrange with the hospital to have it ready and set up by 7 a.m.," he confirmed.

"Thank you! Will that be all Stan needs?" I asked.

"It should be. Just stay home away from people and keep me updated on his condition. We can also liaise with Rochester General Hospital if Stan needs anything more," he said.

The following morning, the last day of 2021, we headed to Westchester Medical Center one last time. Stan got the antibody infusion through an IV. We stayed for another 30 minutes to make sure he doesn't have any reaction to it.

Thankfully it was an easy procedure with no side effects and we were finally cleared to head home.

As I drove out of the big city, I looked over at Stan who had fallen asleep. He looked so peaceful.

"Thank you Papa, thank you for keeping your promise. Thank you that I am not taking this drive alone. Thank you that I can take this drive home WITH my husband," I prayed.

I gently pulled a blanket over his hands to keep him warm. Snowflakes started falling slowly onto the windscreen. The season had changed.

My heart was filled with gratitude as I thought about what we had been through in less than two months. The miracle we had just lived. I felt honored that my God chose us for this journey. That He blessed us the way He did.

CHAPTER 12

Losing Dave Maroney

Our dear friend Mark had looked after everything for us at home and even fixed the bathroom ceiling which Stan didn't get to do before he fell ill.

We didn't want any dust or anything to make him sick with his immune system suppressed. Mark also set up the HEPA filters I had ordered so the air quality in the house would be good for Stan.

By New Year's Eve, we arrived home. What a journey. Not just the road trip but the past few weeks. I put Stan in bed straight away to get his feet up and I started unloading the car.

I was grateful to be able to go into the New Year at home. Later that evening we fell asleep with the sounds of fireworks in the distance.

The next few days were filled with falling back into some kind of routine. Stan was still struggling with fluid retention and became dedicated to walking around the house every day to get his circulation going and to get the water off his legs and feet.

It was painful but he persevered.

On Wednesday, January 12th, Stan and I headed back down to Westchester for another biopsy on the 13th. Harboring Hearts once again blessed us with gas cards as well as a hotel booking for the two nights while in Westchester. They have been angels to us in this time.

Early in the evening we were almost at the hotel when my phone rang. It was Candy. We had spoken regularly since we no longer got to see each other at the hospital but never in a million years would I have ever expected this call.

"Dave died," I heard her say hysterically.

"WHAT?" I yelled. I pulled over straight away as this took the wind out of my sails, and heard Candy crying uncontrollably.

"HOW?" I asked.

The last time we spoke was only a day or two ago and Dave was doing so well. They also spoke about a transfer to rehab.

"His heart stopped. They gave him medication for his anxiety and his heart stopped!" Candy cried.

"Candy, I can't believe this," I said. I was at a loss for words.

"He was doing so well, Liesl," Candy said, struggling to find words through the tears. "They say he is braindead," she continued. "They will confirm tomorrow but there is nothing there, Liesl," Candy said.

I could not believe what I was hearing.

"Candy, I am so sorry, I don't have words. Karen must be beside herself with grief and shock," I said.

"She is a mess, Liesl. We all are. We loved that man so much, He was so good to Karen," Candy continued.

The following day Candy let me know they confirmed there was no brain activity with Dave and he was officially declared braindead.

Dave's mother and family came to the hospital to say their goodbyes and then Karen did the most incredible thing.

She sat down with Dave's mom and asked, "Can we sign Dave up for organ donation?"

"I don't know," his mother replied.

"I have to tell you a story, a true story, about a man I met in this hospital," Karen explained.

She continued telling Dave's mom about her and her mom meeting me and hearing about Stan.

She shared how ill Stan was and how the miracle of receiving a new heart had saved his life, and how well he was doing now. How she saw me going through all the emotions. That Stan would be dead by now if he didn't receive a heart and I would be a widow.

Karen told Dave's mom about how inspired Dave was hearing about Stan and the excitement he showed hearing Stan received a heart.

Dave's mom was touched and she agreed. This is something Dave would have wanted. They signed for Dave to become a hero.

On January 15, 2022, David P. Schultz Maroney took the hero walk. At the bottom end of the hallway Dave's bed appeared around the corner. Almost in slow motion.

The sunlight through the windows lit up the hallway and medical staff filtered from every door lining up to salute Dave.

A few doctors walked along behind the bed, slowly pushing it towards the OR. Behind them was Dave's mom, and a few family members.

Next to the bed, crying uncontrollably, Karen held onto Dave's hand. He was covered in his favorite blanket, his body lifeless.

Karen wanted to capture every memory she could, while Dave was still there, so she asked Candy to record the walk for her. Candy struggled to keep it together.

I could not imagine how hard this was for them both but my heart bled for Candy knowing, as a mother myself, all you want to do is take your child's pain away, but she couldn't.

Karen took every step, her last steps with Dave, all the way to the OR entrance. Here it was the final goodbye. How do you say goodbye to someone who you loved so deeply? Someone who loved you so unconditionally.

God was showing us the grief and process the donor goes through. I could not help but think about Stan's donor and family. This is what they experienced. A tragedy. We had a personal glimpse of what the other side of our miracle looked like.

Never in a million years could we have known Dave was going to become a donor himself. He fought such a battle through all the medical issues and then, right before he was discharged, a tragedy hit.

Stan's donors' selfless act of leaving a heart for Stan had inspired another donor, saving more recipient lives. This amazing donor caused a ripple effect and saved so many more lives. I yearned for Stan's donor and family to know this.

Karen, one day, one day when it is your appointment with God, Dave will be there to welcome you.

I thank Dave for allowing me to meet Candy and Karen and for not just finding new friends but someone who feels like family.
Seeing the impact organ donation makes firsthand changed my viewpoint drastically. I went from a signed-up organ donor to an organ donor advocate.

Personally, I feel that on the day when it is time for me to go be with God when He awaits me with open arms and I hopefully hear the words, "Well done," from Papa, I will leave a body behind which might make an impact on lives like Stan's donor made on us.

Dave saved lives. Although I never met him in person, I believe he was the type of man who would not have wanted it any other way. He was a man with a heart of gold.

Dave Maroney was a hero who became a legend! He will be deeply missed. Thank you, Dave, for showing Karen what love is. Thank you for what you meant to me and Stan. Thank you for what you meant in the lives of those who were saved by receiving your organs.

One day we will meet. In the meantime, we will celebrate your life.

CHAPTER 13

Her Name Was Deedra

As Stan's health increased and we knew what a donor family goes through seeing it from Dave's beautiful girlfriend's viewpoint, we were desperate to know more about Stan's donor.

I contacted LiveOnNY as Dave Gray, the patient advocate, had recommended. I explained to them that Stan had received a heart transplant at Westchester on December 1, 2021.

I received an email back reading, "Hi Liesl. Yes, the donor was registered with us and I can tell you it was a female and she was 43 years old."

"If you would like to write to the family please send it to me and I will see if they are ready to receive a letter," the email continued.

How do you write to a family who lost someone? Someone so selfless that they chose to leave their organs for someone else to live. To have made that decision during one of the most devastating moments in their lives.

How do you thank someone in a situation like this? The words, Thank you, are simply not enough.

We didn't know how she died. How big her family is, if she was married, so many unknowns. Over the next few weeks, Stan and I started putting some thoughts onto paper.

Even when we had finished the letter and changed it so many times it still felt inadequate.

I emailed the letter and two photos to LiveOnNY and asked if they could send it to the family.

"Absolutely, Liesl. What a beautiful letter," Kayla wrote.

"I will ask them if they are ready to receive it and once I send it, I will let you know they have requested it," she continued.

I loved the respect it was all handled with. Not just dumping an email in the donor's family inbox but first asking if they would like to receive an email.

Days went by. Weeks. Then, on Valentine's Day, we received an email from Kayla, "Liesl I wanted to let you know that the donor's husband received the letter today and he said he will also show her mother."

I cried. Again. How hard must this be for this family? We hoped for a response but weeks and months went by. We wanted to know more about her.

We wanted to celebrate her life. Name her when someone asks if we know anything about the donor.

There was nothing we could do but wait. And then, six months later, something amazing happened.

On Wednesday, August 17th, 2022 my dear friend Kim messaged me.

"Hey girl, you are in a funk. Come for coffee tonight, I will set up the ramp at the door. See you at 7 p.m.," the message read.

I had bone fusion surgery on my left foot eight weeks earlier and was not allowed to walk on the foot for yet another two weeks. My frustration levels were through the roof and I was using a knee scooter to get around.

Kim knew I had cabin fever and insisted I come around to her place. We sat talking and her boyfriend Kelly joined in as they asked me if we had contact with the donor family at all.

I told them we wrote a letter and they received it but no response yet. I mentioned that I know it might be too soon for them and we were planning on trying to send another letter around the one year anniversary and would then quit writing if we did not get a response.

We would then accept that they do not want to make contact and as hard as that would be, I would accept it out of respect. Every time I spoke about the incredible gift they gave Stan I became emotional.

Every single time I spoke about the donor I would start crying. I told Kim all I know is the donor was female and 43 years old and she must have passed away within a day or three before Stan got the transplant.

Not many people are aware but when someone is declared brain dead, the day of that confirmation is the official date of death. So someone might be declared dead and only after a couple of days become a donor.

Kim knows me, she knew this was hard for me to not know more about.

"Have you checked obituaries," she asked.

"Oh yes. For hours! I gave up," I said.

"I did too Liesl," she said and explained that she had also stopped looking.

It was great to spend some time with these awesome humans and I felt energized again.

The following morning I woke up to a text from Kim.

"I found her. I will confirm in a minute," it read.

My heart started pounding.

I needed to be sure, 100% sure Kim found the right family.

Then the message from Kim again, "It's her. I found her brother. They got your letter. He wants to speak to you."

I started weeping. I cannot put into words the emotion I felt.

Kim placed the donor's brother and me in a chat room and he asked if he could add her mother as well as her children. Oh Lord, I was a mess. Kids, she had kids?

Stan walked back into the bedroom and was wondering why I was such a mess as he was unaware of the messages from Kim and that we had made contact with the donor family.

"It's your donor's family honey!" I struggled to say as I was crying.

I could see my husband developed tears as he caught up with the conversation.

Deedra Marie Manning was her name.

A forty-three year old lady who left her estranged husband, four children, her mother, her brother and the man she had fallen in love with, a man she was planning on marrying once her divorce was final.

We all spoke for a while and it became clear that they are such an incredible family. Our kind of tribe. The more Stan spoke to Deedra's mother about her and things she would get up to, it was clear that this heart match was more than just a perfect medical match.

There are so many similarities in personality between Stan and Deedra. Mostly, being headstrong. I couldn't help but wonder, is Stan doing so incredibly well because they were so similar on so many levels.

I believe a big part of life that we tend to forget is that we are spiritual beings having a physical experience, not the other way around. The same type of faith I had that Stan would make it through is the type of faith I now have that his body will NEVER go into rejection.

We have adopted Deedra's heart. It is a part of Stan now. His body has accepted it and I believe her heart has now truly become Stan's.

The family have agreed to meet with us later this year which will be yet another blessing. I look forward to hugging her family and thanking them in person for this gift they allowed Deedra to leave behind. A gift that saved Stan's life.

Deedra was in the same hospital as Stan. She was in the Medical ICU and her mother decided to sign her for donation when she was declared brain dead on November 28th, one day after her forty-third birthday.

Deedra's mom, Leda, has been through so much, the entire family has, but my heart bleeds for her mom. To lose a child, I cannot imagine that pain. I find healing in being able to speak to Leda.

I called Candy to share the news and she was so happy for us.

"Candy do you realize that Stan, Dave, and Deedra were in the same ICU at the same time for a couple of days?" I said.

"That is so weird, Liesl," she replied.

"CANDY! Oh, my word! I am sending you a photo of a man right now. Do you recognize this man?" I asked.

Candy was confused until she received the photo.

"Oh my gosh, yes! He was at the ICU!" she said.

"Exactly! I have goosebumps. Do you remember one day we were standing outside the MICU ringing the bell, Me, you, Karen, and this man!" I said.

"YES! Who is this?" she asked.

"That is Deedra's estranged husband!' I said and felt goosebumps from my head to my toes.

This is the man I walked behind after they opened the doors and I saw him go into one of the ICU rooms.

There was a lady in the bed. It was Deedra. I saw Stan's donor not realizing this is the woman who will save my husband's life in a few days. I was moving past Deedra's room and her family for a few days before Stan was moved to Cardiac ICU.

This was so much to wrap my mind around. Stan was simply God-smacked and could not utter a word.

God's details were overwhelming. Details we were now becoming aware of, almost nine months after the transplant.

It felt like our roller coaster had come to a stop and the only thing remaining was to meet Deedra's family. We plan on doing this early December when Stan will be back at Westchester for his one year medical checkup.

A special meeting where everyone who loved her can once again hear her heart beating. Her heart which Stan has now adopted.

So with our roller coaster feeling like it came to a standstill…Did we enjoy the ride? This is not a ride you get off saying, "Wow, let's do that again." This is a ride that changes how you see life. That changes your intimate relationship with God.

It gives you hope. Peace. It leaves you in awe of God's mercy and that He has a plan for each of us just like it says in Jeremiah 29:11. "'For I know the plans I have for you', declares the Lord, 'plans to prosper you and not to harm you, plans to give you hope and a future'."

Most of all it reminds you that this life is a short time on this planet and eternity waits in Heaven. This journey gave us a look how different yet intertwined our journeys could be. How God orchestrates every action. The experience for myself was vastly different from what it was for Stan.

I experienced the stress of being an advocate, being aware of every little detail while Stan finds it hard to remember certain things to this day.

Of the actual transplant day, he has almost no recollection. Maybe that is a blessing.

This was a very tough journey for both of us in a very different way. Would I change it? NO! My husband is alive.

I thank God for this incredible journey. A journey we would never have chosen but God gave us no option and in the process, He fulfilled His promise.

"I am going to perform a miracle in Stan's life, I am not done with Him yet."

This experience has changed my husband. He has become a better man and a better husband. A better person. I am excited to see how Papa continues to work in Stan's life.

There is a Bible verse that became a very real verse in our lives…

Ezekiel 36:26

I will give you a new heart and put a new spirit in you; I will remove from you your heart of stone and give you a heart of flesh.

God gave Stan a new heart and He put a new spirit within him. How can anyone doubt this living God?

How can anyone hear this miraculous story and still not believe in the power of Jesus?

If you are one of those people… I have one thing to say to you. **God is not done with you yet!**

ORGAN DONATION

We hope this story has inspired you to sign up as an organ donor. You could become the hero in many people's lives. You could become a Deedra in someone's life. That day she chose to sign up as an organ donor she could not have imagined how she would one day change our lives.

One donor can save up to 8 lives while up to 75 lives can be changed through tissue donation. A person is added to the National transplant waiting list every 10 minutes.

In New York State alone 9000 people are awaiting organs. 1 New Yorker dies every day waiting for a life-saving transplant.

You are never too old to sign up and no, it doesn't mean the doctors are not going to do everything in their power to save you if you are a donor.

It makes it so much easier on your family if a tragedy happens to know that was your wishes, and it doesn't become a decision they have to make.

Get signed up at your local DMV and get a driver's license that shows you are a donor or register now at **www.donatelife.net/register**

To assist Harboring Hearts in supporting families of transplant from out of town in NYC area, please visit **www.HarboringHearts.org**

It is organizations like this who make such an incredible impact on people in their darkest hours. Thank you again to everyone at Harboring Hearts.

AFTERWORD

I pray this book has inspired you in some way to NEVER give up. NEVER to lose HOPE!

If you find yourself on a roller-coaster, SURRENDER. Give the situation to God. Totally! Not just Jesus take the wheel, but Jesus take the wheel and let me get into the back seat.

Stop trying to control what you cannot control and give it to God. Allow Him to perform miracles in your life.

To the many people we have met online and in person who are awaiting organs on transplant lists, do not give up. Your miracle could happen tomorrow.

To every single person who has not signed up for organ donation, do it now. Please. One day there will be a Stan waiting on life and your selfless act might save not just a life but lives! Maybe one day one of YOUR loved ones might need a lifesaving organ.

ABOUT THE AUTHOR

Liesl is a South African-born and raised public speaker and ex-strongwoman.

She published a book called "Warrior Within" in 2020 about her challenges as a child and how she found the inner strength to keep going.

Her passion is working with those who have lost hope. She can encourage the hopeless to pick themselves up and fight another day.

She is a woman of God and speaks about His miracles to everyone she meets.

In 2019 she immigrated to the USA. Her daughter, Zaan, and her husband, Taylor, also live in New York. Her son, Duncan, lives in Cape Town, South Africa.

Liesl married Stan in 2020 after they met in 2017. They live in Upstate NY, near Rochester.

"To God be ALL the Glory. He is a God of miracles. A God who keeps His promises. He is my provider, my everything.

I am forever grateful to Papa for giving me more time with my husband." ~ Liesl Schoonraad

www.ingramcontent.com/pod-product-compliance
Lightning Source LLC
Chambersburg PA
CBHW031609210526
45464CB00004B/1497